Glucose Regulation

Editor

CELIA LEVESQUE

NURSING CLINICS
OF NORTH AMERICA

www.nursing.theclinics.com

Consulting Editor
STEPHEN D. KRAU

December 2017 • Volume 52 • Number 4

ELSEVIER

1600 John F. Kennedy Boulevard • Suite 1800 • Philadelphia, Pennsylvania, 19103-2899

http://www.theclinics.com

NURSING CLINICS OF NORTH AMERICA Volume 52, Number 4
December 2017 ISSN 0029-6465, ISBN-13: 978-0-323-55284-4

Editor: Kerry Holland
Developmental Editor: Casey Potter

Nursing Clinics of North America (ISSN 0029-6465) is published quarterly by Elsevier Inc., 360 Park Avenue South, New York, NY 10010-1710. Months of issue are March, June, September, and December. Periodicals postage paid at New York, NY and additional mailing offices. Subscription price per year is, $155.00 (US individuals), $465.00 (US institutions), $275.00 (international individuals), $567.00 (international institutions), $220.00 (Canadian individuals), $567.00 (Canadian institutions), $100.00 (US students), and $135.00 (international students). To receive student/resident rate, orders must be accompanied by name of affiliated institution, date of term, and the signature of program/residency coordinator on institution letterhead. Orders will be billed at individual rate until proof of status is received. Foreign air speed delivery is included in all *Clinics* subscription prices. All prices are subject to change without notice. **POSTMASTER:** Send address changes to *Nursing Clinics*, Elsevier Health Sciences Division, Subscription Customer Service, 3251 Riverport Lane, Maryland Heights, MO 63043. **Customer Service: Telephone: 1-800-654-2452** (U.S. and Canada); **1-314-447-8871 (outside U.S. and Canada). Fax: 1-314-447-8029. E-mail: journalscustomerservice-usa@elsevier.com** (for print support) and **journalsonlinesupport-usa@elsevier.com** (for online support).

Nursing Clinics of North America is covered in *EMBASE/Excerpta Medica, MEDLINE/PubMed (Index Medicus), Social Sciences Citation Index, Current Contents, ASCA, Cumulative Index to Nursing, RNdex Top 100,* and Allied Health Literature and International Nursing Index (INI).

Contributors

CONSULTING EDITOR

STEPHEN D. KRAU, PhD, RN, CNE
Associate Professor, Vanderbilt University Medical Center, School of Nursing, Nashville, Tennessee

EDITOR

CELIA LEVESQUE, RN, MSN, CNS-BC, NP-C, CDE, BC-ADM
Advanced Practice Provider, Department of Endocrine Neoplasia and Hormonal Disorders, The University of Texas MD Anderson Cancer Center, Houston, Texas

AUTHORS

JANE A. ANDERSON, PhD, RN, FNP-C, FAAN
Health Sciences Research and Development Center for Innovations in Quality, Effectiveness and Safety (IQUEST), Michael E. DeBakey VA Medical Center (MEDVAMC), Houston, Texas

VERONICA J. BRADY, PhD, MSN, FNP-BC, BC-ADM, CDE
Diabetes Nurse Practitioner, University of Nevada, Reno School of Medicine, Reno, Nevada

ANNE KAY BRINKMAN, MSN, APRN, A-GNP-C
Advanced Practice Registered Nurse, Department of Endocrine Neoplasia and Hormonal Disorders, The University of Texas MD Anderson Cancer Center, Houston, Texas

KATE CRAWFORD, RN, MSN, ANP-C, BC-ADM
Nurse Practitioner, North Texas Endocrine Center, Dallas, Texas

SELIECE DODDS, MSN, ACNS-BC, APRN, CDE
Advanced Practice Provider, Division of Internal Medicine, Department of Endocrine Neoplasia and Hormonal Disorders, The University of Texas MD Anderson Cancer Center, Houston, Texas

ANN L. HORGAS, RN, PhD, FGSA, FAAN
Associate Professor, University of Florida College of Nursing, Gainesville, Florida

CELIA LEVESQUE, RN, MSN, CNS-BC, NP-C, CDE, BC-ADM
Advanced Practice Provider, Department of Endocrine Neoplasia and Hormonal Disorders, The University of Texas MD Anderson Cancer Center, Houston, Texas

JOHN E. MBUE, PharmD, MS, BCOP
Michael E. DeBakey VA Medical Center (MEDVAMC), Houston, Texas

NGOZI D. MBUE, PhD, RN, ANP-C
Advanced Post-Doctoral Fellow, Health Sciences Research and Development Center for Innovations in Quality, Effectiveness and Safety (IQUEST), Michael E. DeBakey VA Medical Center (MEDVAMC), Baylor College of Medicine, Houston, Texas

DEBORAH L. MCCREA, MSN, RN, FNP-BC, CNS, CEN, CFRN, EMT-P
Instructor, Clinical Nursing, Department of Acute and Continuing Care, The University of Texas Health Science Center at Houston, School of Nursing, Houston, Texas

MARJORIE R. ORTIZ, RN, MSN, AGPCNP-BC
Advanced Practice Registered Nurse, Department of Endocrine Neoplasia and Hormonal Disorders, The University of Texas MD Anderson Cancer Center, Houston, Texas

SIGI VARGHESE, RN, MSN, FNP-C, BC-ADM
Department of Endocrine Neoplasia and Hormonal Disorders, The University of Texas MD Anderson Cancer Center, Houston, Texas

MARA LYNN WILSON, RN, MS, FNP-C, CDE
Family Nurse Practitioner, Department of Endocrine Neoplasia and Hormonal Disorders, The University of Texas MD Anderson Cancer Center, Houston, Texas

JESSICA K. YAKUSH WILLIAMS, MSPAS, PA-C
Department of Endocrine Neoplasia and Hormonal Disorders, The University of Texas MD Anderson Cancer Center, Houston, Texas

Contents

mellitus, as the disease progresses, it may become a necessary addition to treatment. The goal of this article is to discuss insulin therapies that are currently available for use in the management of diabetes, from the old to the new and novel, and briefly discuss insulin use in special populations.

An estimated 1 million people use an insulin pump to manage their diabetes. Few medical professionals understand or feel comfortable caring for people who use an insulin pump. This article helps the medical professional understand the reasons why the insulin pump helps the user to achieve better glycemic control, have more flexibility, and enjoy a better quality of life. Additionally, this article discusses the advantages, disadvantages, candidate selection, contraindications, basic functions, and troubleshooting of the insulin pump.

Hypoglycemia is a common problem in patients with diabetes, and often limits those trying to achieve tight glucose control. Achieving optimal glucose control is necessary to prevent microvascular complications. Hypoglycemia can cause mild disturbances to daily life, but in severe cases can be fatal. Patient education of hypoglycemic medications, risk factors, contributing factors, and prevention strategies should be included in the care plan of patients at risk of developing hypoglycemia.

Diabetes mellitus is a leading cause of chronic kidney disease, prompting the need for monitoring and management of this complex condition in those diagnosed with diabetes. Management is often multifaceted and includes lifestyle modification, management of hyperglycemia, and management of hypertension and hyperlipidemia to slow progression of kidney disease and to mitigate cardiovascular risks associated with diabetes and kidney disease. This article reviews the current literature regarding monitoring and management of diabetic kidney disease and chronic kidney disease in diabetes.

Diabetes is a common chronic illness in children and adolescents. This article discusses the prevalence, diagnostic criteria, types, treatment, and transition of care into adulthood.

Abnormal lipids, sometimes referred to as diabetes dyslipidemia, is a common condition in patients with diabetes. With the increasing number of patients with abnormal lipids, especially those with type 2 diabetes, health care practitioners, including nurses, must properly manage patients with diabetes as well as abnormal lipids. This article examines the pathophysiology of abnormal lipids, the management of abnormal lipids, and the lipid goals for patients with diabetes. Last, this article discusses pharmacologic and nonpharmacologic therapies and the role of primary care providers and nurses in the management of abnormal lipids.

Diabetes is a complex medical condition that requires evidence-based care. This article discusses the current diabetes screening, diagnostic criteria, and treatment recommendations for patients with type 1 diabetes, type 2 diabetes, gestational diabetes, and prediabetes.

Prediabetes is a complex multifactorial metabolic disorder that extends beyond glucose control. Current studies have found that microvascular disease (neuropathy, nephropathy, and retinopathy), macrovascular disease (stroke, coronary artery disease, and peripheral vascular disease), periodontal disease, cognitive dysfunction, blood pressure changes, obstructive sleep apnea, low testosterone level, fatty liver disease, and cancer are some of conditions that are present with the onset of glycemic dysregulation. The presence of prediabetes increases the risk of developing type 2 diabetes 3-fold to 10-fold. The identification and treatment of prediabetes are imperative to prevent or delay the progression to type 2 diabetes.

Diabetes mellitus is a common chronic disease affecting approximately 9% of the US population. Successful management of diabetes demands constant self-management on the part of the patient. The patient must balance diabetes medications, blood glucose monitoring, food intake, physical activity, and management of diabetes-related acute and chronic complications. The patient is often bombarded with misinformation from friends, relatives, and such sources as the Internet and social media. This article discusses the current recommendations for diabetes self-management education and skills including medical nutrition therapy, physical activity, smoking cessation, and assessment for diabetes distress.

Special Article

Treating pain in older adults can be complex because of the age-related physiologic changes, comorbidities, and polypharmacy. Thus, an individualized, multimodal treatment approach is recommended. Treatment plans should include pharmacologic and nonpharmacologic strategies. Several important clinical guidelines and expert panel statements are available to guide health care providers in the best practices for treating pain in older adults. This article provides evidence-based recommendations for pharmacological and non-pharmacological pain management in older adults.

NURSING CLINICS OF
NORTH AMERICA

Foreword

Diabetes: A Health Threat on the Rise

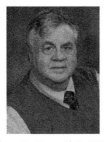

Stephen D. Krau, PhD, RN, CNE
Consulting Editor

The content in this issue provides nurses with an essential "handbook" on glucose regulation and diabetes. The prevalence and predicted growth of diabetes are well supported. Currently, diabetes is the most common metabolic disorder worldwide, and the incidence among adults in the United States continues to grow. There is clear evidence that the incidence of diabetes will continue to grow worldwide. Along with the disease itself, the associated health burden is expected to grow substantially as well. These increases are attributed to rapid developments and subsequent changes in lifestyle, and the comparatively slow growth of health care systems. Diabetes and its multisystem complications are predicted to be high in the United States and especially high in low- and middle-income countries worldwide.[1] The highest increases in the prevalence of the disease are anticipated to occur in Asia, the Middle East, and Africa, where it is predicted that there will be a 50% increase by 2030.[2]

Type 1 and type 2 diabetes have different causes and characteristics, but both are diabetes and are clinically characterized by hyperglycemia due to chronic and/or relative insulin insufficiency.[2] The cause of type 1 diabetes is considered hyperglycemia that occurs as a result of a complex disease process whereby genetic and environmental factors lead to an autoimmune response that still is not completely understood. During this process, the pancreatic beta-cells within the islets of Langerhans are destroyed. This creates a condition in which individuals must rely on exogenous insulin for glucose control and actual survival.

The majority of diabetic cases are type 2, which comprise about 85% of diabetic cases. "In this form of the disease, peripheral insulin resistance and compensatory hypersecretion of insulin from the pancreatic islets may precede the decline in islet secretory function."[2] Reduced insulin sensitivity is most conspicuously demonstrated in skeletal muscle, liver, and adipose tissue. The causes of type 2 diabetes are thought to be the result of environmental factors rather than only genetic factors. "It remains

Nurs Clin N Am 52 (2017) ix–x
https://doi.org/10.1016/j.cnur.2017.09.002
0029-6465/17/© 2017 Published by Elsevier Inc.

nursing.theclinics.com

unlikely that genetic factors or ageing per se alone can explain this dramatic increase in the prevalence of type 2 diabetes."[2]

The complications associated with diabetes impact every system of the body. As vascular changes are inherent in uncontrolled diabetes, directly or indirectly every organ is affected. The ultimate goal of diabetes management is to prevent or reverse the vascular complications so prevalent in persons with diabetes. It is essential that health care professionals understand the mechanisms that lead to disease development and progression, but also how these alterations evolve through a temporal manner. Concurrent to glucose regulation, it is important to consider appropriate management of patient obesity, hyperlipidemia, and hypertension. "This is particularly important given that a number of previous studies have shown reduced efficacy of the various interventions, once the disease has progressed beyond a certain point."[2]

Stephen D. Krau, PhD, RN, CNE
Vanderbilt University Medical Center
309 Godchaux, 461 21st Avenue South
Nashville, TN 37240, USA

E-mail address:
steve.krau@vanderbilt.edu

REFERENCES

1. Guariguata L, Whiting DR, Hambleton I, et al. Global estimates of diabetes prevalence for 2013 and projections for 2035. Diabetes Res Clin Pract 2014;103:137–49.
2. Forbes JM, Cooper ME. Mechanisms of diabetic complications. Physiol Rev 2013; 93:137–8.

Preface

Glucose Regulation

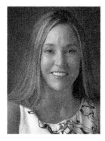

Celia Levesque, RN, MSN, CNS-BC, NP-C, CDE, BC-ADM
Editor

Nursing plays an important role in the care and education of the patient with diabetes. Diabetes mellitus is a costly chronic disease affecting millions worldwide. The cost of diabetes is measured not only in terms of money but also in terms of acute and chronic diabetes-related complications, and quality and quantity of life. Diabetes not only affects the patient, but also affects the patient's significant others. Diabetes is largely a self-managed disease; therefore, the patient must learn how to correctly perform self-care. The nurse needs to know the current recommendations in order to effectively care for and educate the patient. This issue discusses the current diabetes standards of care based on the American Diabetes Association and American Association of Clinical Endocrinologist recommendations. Other topics, discussed in detail, include management of prediabetes, type 1 diabetes, type 2 diabetes, diabetes medications, insulin pump therapy, therapeutic lifestyle recommendations, management of hyperlipidemia, chronic kidney disease, hypoglycemia, and management of diabetes in children.

Celia Levesque, RN, MSN, CNS-BC, NP-C, CDE, BC-ADM
Department of Endocrine Neoplasia and Hormonal Disorders
MD Anderson Cancer Center
1515 Holcomb Boulevard
Houston, TX 77030, USA

E-mail address:
clevesqu@mdanderson.org

Nurs Clin N Am 52 (2017) xi
https://doi.org/10.1016/j.cnur.2017.09.001
0029-6465/17/© 2017 Published by Elsevier Inc.

Management of Type 1 Diabetes

Anne Kay Brinkman, MSN, APRN, A-GNP-C

KEYWORDS

- Type 1 diabetes • Glucose management • Insulin therapy • Autoimmune • Nursing

KEY POINTS

- Differentiation between type 1 and other types of diabetes is an integral part of competent nursing care.
- Immune related cancer therapy has been identified as a new and emerging causality for type 1 diabetes.
- Nurses are an important part of the diabetes care team and should be aware of diabetes complications.
- Insulin therapy options are expanding with the addition of new preparations.
- Mortality related to cardiovascular disease in type 1 diabetic patients remains higher than the general population.
- Close follow up with expert medical specialists is important in early detection and treatment of diabetes related complications.

INTRODUCTION

Type 1 diabetes, although much rarer than type 2 diabetes, is also becoming more prevalent. More is known about the possible causes of type 1 diabetes, and strategies to prevent the evolution of the disease are being developed. Clinicians should be aware of these changes and the current standards of care to provide complete care for patients with type 1 diabetes. This article discusses the epidemiology, pathophysiology, diagnosis, management strategies, and long-term outcomes of patients with type 1 diabetes.

EPIDEMIOLOGY

In the United States, an estimated 3 million individuals have type 1 diabetes.[1] Type 1 diabetes has been classically known as a childhood disease, with the peak age of diagnosis in the mid teenage years.[2] However, the larger proportion of individuals

Disclosure Statement: The author has nothing to disclose.
Department of Endocrine Neoplasia and Hormonal Disorders, UT MD Anderson Cancer Center, 1400 Pressler Street, Unit 1461, Houston, TX 77030, USA
E-mail address: AKBrinkman@mdanderson.org

Nurs Clin N Am 52 (2017) 499–511
http://dx.doi.org/10.1016/j.cnur.2017.07.001
0029-6465/17/© 2017 Elsevier Inc. All rights reserved.

with type 1 diabetes are adults who have been living with diabetes since childhood or were diagnosed during adulthood.[1]

In the United States, type 1 diabetes accounts for 5% of all diabetes cases in adults.[2] The incidence of type 1 diabetes is increasing at a rate of 3% to 5% per year based on studies reviewed from the United States, Germany, Poland, and Italy.[3] There are several theories as to why this disease, considered primarily autoimmune related, is increasing in frequency. It is well established that genetic predisposition is a major factor in a person's risk of type 1 diabetes development; however, the increasing incidence suggests additional contributing factors. Researchers are exploring how a combination of genetic predisposition and interaction with environmental factors is responsible for the increasing rate of type 1 diabetes. Research is currently evaluating various environmental factors and how they may be influencing the development of diabetes. Infection, diet and body size, pollutants, gut flora, vitamin D exposure, geographic location, insulin resistance, and prenatal environment are all factors that are theorized to increase the risk of type 1 diabetes development; however, not all studies have found clear supportive evidence.[3]

PATHOPHYSIOLOGY

Most type 1 diabetes develops when the immune system attacks and destroys pancreatic β cells. This process results in progressive insulin deficiency leading to complete dependence on exogenous insulin.[2] Autoimmune markers can be detected in the blood of patients with this type of diabetes and can also be used for early detection of at risk family members. These markers include islet cell autoantibodies and autoantibodies to glutamic acid decarboxylase, insulin, protein tyrosine phosphatases (IA-2 and IA-2β), and zinc transporter protein (ZnT8).[4] The destruction of β cells can occur rapidly, as is typically seen in childhood diabetes, or more slowly leading to insulin dependence in adulthood.

Over the last decade, immune checkpoint inhibitors have been approved for the treatment of several cancers. Although rarely reported, new-onset type 1 diabetes is a rare side effect of some of these therapies. Recent review of case reports identified patients who presented with type 1 diabetes anywhere from 1 week to 7 months after initial treatment. In this review, some patients were found to have autoantibodies associated with type 1 diabetes whereas others were antibody negative.[5] Further research is needed to determine whether this variation of type 1 diabetes will be permanent and whether it should be treated differently than traditional type 1 diabetes.

Idiopathic type 1 diabetes is defined by periods of absence of insulin production without the presence of β-cell autoimmunity. This form of type 1 diabetes is strongly inherited and occurs most frequently in patients with African or Asian ancestry. The episodic nature of this disease put these patients at increased risk for diabetic ketoacidosis, and their insulin replacement requirements may vary or be intermittent.[4]

DIAGNOSIS

Differentiating between type 1 and 2 diabetes is important so that the patient can be optimally treated. The diagnosis should be made with a combination of data including clinical presentation, laboratory data, and family history. Ongoing re-evaluation of the diagnosis may be needed for patients who do not respond as expected to prescribed treatments.

Current criteria for the diagnosis of diabetes, based on the American Diabetes Association (ADA) Standards for Medical Care 2017 Guidelines, do not differentiate between type 1 and type 2 diabetes, and include[1]:

- Hemoglobin A1c greater than 6.5%
- Fasting glucose greater than 126 mg/dL
- Two-hour postprandial glucose ≥200 mg/dL during the oral glucose tolerance test
- Random plasma glucose ≥200 mg/dL in a patient with classic symptoms of hyperglycemia or hyperglycemic crisis

In children with type 1 diabetes, the diagnosis is generally made at the time of symptomatic presentation with high random blood glucose values and classic symptoms of severe hyperglycemia such as polyuria, polydipsia, and ketonemia. The hemoglobin A1c is assessed, but the purpose is generally to determine the duration of hyperglycemia rather than to establish the diagnosis itself.[4]

In adult patients, the onset may be more gradual, and therefore patients may receive an incorrect diagnosis of type 2 diabetes. The ADA recommends that clinicians consider the possibility of type 1 diabetes in newly diagnosed type 2 diabetics who have persistent hyperglycemia after treatment with noninsulin agents.[1]

In addition to the typical baseline laboratory evaluation for newly diagnosed diabetes, measurement of pancreatic autoantibodies can be useful in differentiating type 1 from type 2 diabetes. Laboratories using highly sensitive measurement techniques can detect nearly 100% of individuals with autoantibodies at diagnosis; however, commercial laboratories may have less reliable techniques; therefore, false-negative results can occur.[1] The surrogate marker for insulin secretion, C-peptide, can also be used as part of the laboratory evaluation. Clinicians should be aware that residual, although typically low, C-peptide may be detected for decades after initial diagnosis.[1]

Family history may also provide clues as to the likelihood of a type 1 diabetes diagnosis. Patients who have a first-degree relative with type 1 diabetes have 15 times the risk of disease development when compared with the general population. In fact, first-degree relatives who are screened and show 2 or more persistent autoantibodies have the highest risk for type 1 diabetes development.[6] Data from a prospective cohort study of children in Colorado, Finland, and Germany showed that children with 2 or more of the previously mentioned autoantibodies had a 70% risk for type 1 diabetes development within 10 years.[6] Factors such as the age of detection, along with other variables, can help predict how quickly the patient may progress to insulin deficiency and diabetes.[4]

Research gathered from first-degree relatives of patients with type 1 diabetes has shown that development of type 1 diabetes occurs in stages (**Fig. 1**). This realization has enabled the potential for earlier detection and further efforts to find a way to prevent or slow the progression of islet cell destruction.[4]

Patients in stage 1 of type 1 diabetes have no symptoms, and their glucose level is normal despite the presence of autoantibodies. In stage 2, patients remain asymptomatic but show early dysglycemia that is still below the criteria for diagnosis of diabetes. Once the patient has progressed to stage 3, they will have symptoms and meet the general criteria for diagnosis of diabetes.[4]

There are no standardized recommendations for screening the family members at risk for type 1 diabetes. The ADA does however recommend that clinicians consider referring first-degree relatives to clinical research studies for antibody testing. Patients

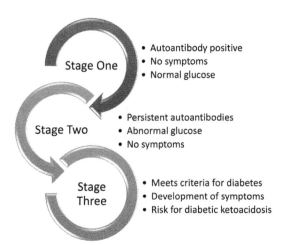

Fig. 1. Stages of type 1 diabetes.

who are found to have antibodies should receive counseling regarding the symptoms of diabetes and have proper follow-up evaluation, as outlined below.[4]

INITIAL EVALUATION

The ADA recommends that individuals with type 1 diabetes have access to clinicians with specific expertise in type 1 diabetes management such as endocrinologists, registered dieticians, diabetes educators, and other specialists as directed by the patient's health needs.[4] The initial evaluation for a patient newly diagnosed with type 1 diabetes should include confirmation of the diagnosis, engagement of the patient in their care plan with appropriate referral to diabetes education programs, screening for early signs of microvascular and macrovascular complications and risk factors for the same, and planning for ongoing care. The general recommendations for initial laboratory evaluation include hemoglobin A1c, fasting lipid profile, liver function tests, serum creatinine, thyroid-stimulating hormone, and spot urinary albumin/creatinine ratio.[4]

MANAGEMENT GOALS

The ADA provides general guidelines for management goals in diabetes, which should be adjusted based on individual patient presentation. The general management goals based on the ADA Standards of Medical Care in Diabetes are listed below[4]:

- Hemoglobin A1c less than 7%
- Blood pressure less than 140/80 mm Hg
- Low-density lipoprotein cholesterol less than 100 mg/dL, triglycerides less than 150 mg/dL, high-density lipoprotein cholesterol greater than 40 mg/dL for men, high-density lipoprotein cholesterol greater than 50 mg/dL for women
- Achievement and maintenance of body weight goals
- Delay or prevention of diabetes complications

Glucose Goals

The hemoglobin A1c test is used to determine the average glucose level of a 2- to 3-month period and is found to accurately predict the risk for complications from diabetes. Monitoring of hemoglobin A1c is recommended at diagnosis and during ongoing care. In general, the ADA recommends monitoring hemoglobin A1c every 3 months in diabetic patients; however, more frequent evaluation may be needed for select patients, such as pregnant women with type 1 diabetes.[7]

In some cases the hemoglobin A1c is not interpretable, such as in conditions that alter the integrity of red blood cells (anemias, hemoglobinopathies, recent blood transfusions). In these cases, fructosamine may be used as a substitute to provide average glucose estimates over a period of about 2 weeks. Fructosamine is also subject to inaccuracy with certain health conditions that alter the serum albumin levels, such as nephrotic syndrome or severe liver disease.[8]

The Diabetes Control and Complications Trial (DCCT) was a landmark clinical trial that showed that type 1 diabetics who were able to achieve hemoglobin A1c values of less than 7% had a significantly lower rate of microvascular complications.[9] The benefit of this level of glucose control was then further supported by a follow-up study of the cohorts from the DCCT, which showed that even if glycemic control worsened over time, those that were previously well controlled still had fewer microvascular and cardiovascular complications when compared with control groups.[10] Therefore, the primary goal of type 1 diabetes management is tight glucose control. The ADA does recognize that each patient's situation is unique, however, and recommends modifying glucose goals based on factors such as age, comorbidities, and hypoglycemic awareness.

ADA Glycemic goals for the management of adults diabetes[1]:

- Hemoglobin A1c less than 7% for health adults
- Hemoglobin A1c less than 7.5% for healthy older adults
- Hemoglobin A1c less than 8% for older adults with intermediate health problems
- Hemoglobin A1c less than 8.5% for older adults with poor health

Glucose Monitoring

Self-monitoring of blood glucose (SMBG) allows a patient to evaluate their own glucose response to both pharmacologic and nonpharmacologic interventions such as exercise and diet. Patients with type 1 diabetes should be educated and evaluated on proper technique and given clear instruction on the frequency of testing, which can commonly be up to 6 to 10 times per day (**Fig. 2**).[4]

The ADA does acknowledge that the use of continuous glucose monitoring (CGM) in adult patients with type 1 diabetes who are on intensive insulin regimens can be beneficial. CGM devices use a small wire inserted under the skin to monitor the glucose found in the interstitial fluid. The information is then transmitted to a receiver device, where it can be viewed as a glucose reading and be used to show trends in glucose levels.[11] The CGM tool has been useful in decreasing hemoglobin A1c results by about 0.5% in adult patients and reducing the frequency of hypoglycemic episodes when compared with SMBG alone.[12] The CGM devices must still be calibrated by traditional finger stick blood glucose values, but in December 2016, the Dexcom G5 (Dexcom, Inc, San Diego, CA, USA) system received approval from the US Food and Drug Administration allowing the use of their CGM to make treatment decisions, whereas previously a finger stick glucose value to confirm CGM data was recommended before treating a glucose value.[11]

The glucose monitoring techniques described previously all have limitations. Clinicians should use a combination of hemoglobin A1c values, SMBG, and CGM data at each appointment to guide treatment decisions.

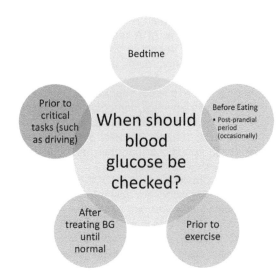

Fig. 2. Frequency of SMBG recommended for type 1 diabetic patients.

PHARMACOLOGIC STRATEGIES

Generally type 1 diabetes is managed with insulin therapy. The initial approach to dosing is weight based with a range of 0.4 to 1.0 U/kg/d of insulin, which is adjusted by confounding factors such as severity of hyperglycemia at presentation, age, and hormonal state.[13] This calculation gives an estimation of the total daily insulin requirement, which is divided into basal and prandial/correction doses. Initially, the recommendation is for 50% of the total daily insulin dose to be given as basal insulin and the remaining 50% divided into mealtime doses.[13] This type of insulin plan is called basal-bolus therapy and is the gold standard for treatment of type 1 diabetes.

Before the acceptance of this standard of therapy, twice-daily dosing with regular insulin and neutral protamine Hagedorn (NPH) insulin were used in what is referred to as *conventional insulin therapy*. This regimen often leads to fluctuation between high and low blood sugar because of greater difficulty anticipating the onset, peak, and duration of action. This type of therapy is not recommended except in circumstances in which the patient is unable to obtain or use rapid-acting/basal insulins.[13]

Prandial Insulin

Mealtime rapid-acting insulin is injected primarily to cover carbohydrates during mealtime but is also used for corrections of elevated blood sugar. The ADA recommends that type 1 diabetes be treated with rapid-acting insulin analogs rather than short-acting insulin (regular) because of increased risk for hypoglycemia with short-acting insulin.[1] Short-acting, regular insulin is the only insulin that can be given through intravenous infusion. Prandial insulins currently available include:

- Lispro (Humalog [Eli Lilly and Company, Indianapolis, IN, USA]); rapid acting
- Aspart (Novolog [Novo Nordisk, Bagsvaerd, Denmark]); rapid acting
- Glulisine (Apidra [Sanofi-Aventis U.S. LLC, Bridgewater, NJ, USA]); rapid acting
- Regular insulin; short acting

The mealtime dose of insulin is further defined by using an insulin/carbohydrate ratio (I:C ratio). The I:C ratio can vary greatly among patients and is determined by having the patient keep a diary over several days documenting insulin doses, glucose values before and 2 to 3 hours after eating, and carbohydrates consumed with associated time stamps.[13]

Basal Insulin

Long-acting basal insulin is injected 1 or 2 times daily. The duration of action of each formulation is different, ranging from 14 to now more than 24 hours with newer insulin formulations. Initially, patients should be started on once-daily dosing, and if this is inadequate, clinicians may consider increasing to twice-daily dosing while using glargine or detemir insulins. Basal insulin adjustments are based on fasting glucose values, with a goal of achieving the target glucose without causing premeal or nocturnal hypoglycemia.[13] The currently available long-acting insulins are listed below.

- Glargine (Lantus [Sanofi-Aventis U.S. LLC, Bridgewater, NJ, USA], Tujeo [Sanofi-Aventis U.S. LLC, Bridgewater, NJ, USA], Basaglar [Eli Lilly and Company, Indianapolis, IN, USA]); long acting
- Detemir (Levemir [Novo Nordisk, Bagsvaerd, Denmark]); long acting
- Degludec (Tresiba [Novo Nordisk, Bagsvaerd, Denmark]); very long acting

Insulin Pump Therapy

Several studies compared multiple daily injections of insulin with insulin pump therapy in patients with type 1 diabetes. The results showed an average decrease of hemoglobin A1c of 0.4% to 0.5% without increasing the frequency of hypoglycemia.[13] The ADA recommends considering insulin pump therapy for motivated adults with type 1 diabetes.[4] Patients should receive specific education regarding insulin pumps and close follow-up to make adjustments to therapy.

Inhaled Insulin

Inhaled insulin is also available for use in type 1 diabetes. The onset of action of the currently available inhaled insulin, Afrezza, is similar to that of injected rapid-acting insulin. Investigative trials found that inhaled insulin is noninferior to rapid-acting injected insulins; however, A1c reductions are greater with injectable insulin.[14] That data, along with the added expense of the medication and the requirement for pulmonary screening, make inhaled insulin as less-attractive option for treatment of type 1 diabetes in most cases.

Adjunctive Therapies

Aside from insulin, pramlintide, an amylin analog manufactured by AstraZeneca Pharmaceuticals (Wilmington, DE, USA) as SymlinPen, has been approved for use in type 1 and type 2 diabetes. The medication slows gastric emptying and therefore delays the absorption of carbohydrates, which can reduce mealtime insulin requirements. The SymlinPen package insert describes common side effects include nausea and early satiety, which can be helpful in weight loss. Studies found a potential hemoglobin A1c reduction of about 0.3% to 0.4%. Clinicians who discuss this therapy with their type 1 diabetic patients should be careful to discuss and plan to reduce mealtime insulin doses to prevent hypoglycemia. Per the SymlinPen prescribing information, mealtime insulin doses should be decreased by 50% on initiation of SymlinPen, and close blood sugar monitoring is advised.[15]

TREATMENT OF THE HOSPITALIZED TYPE 1 DIABETIC

Treatment of individuals with type 1 diabetes in the acute care setting often differs greatly from the care required by type 2 diabetics. Clinicians should be aware that type 1 diabetics may have difficulty with fasting requirements and may need more intensive glucose monitoring and modifications to existing insulin therapy. Patients with type 1 diabetes are considered at high risk for hypoglycemia during periods of fasting and for diabetic ketoacidosis if their basal insulin is not administered. Nurses and all members of the care team should be aware that basal insulin should not be held without specific indication.[1]

Patients using insulin pumps should be allowed to continue to use their pump as long as they are alert and oriented and able to self-manage the device. Use of insulin pumps are contraindicated in critically ill or unstable patients. Staff and patients should also be aware that insulin pumps must be removed before entering areas in close proximity to MRI.[13]

Complications

Hypoglycemia is an unfortunate and likely complication of intensive glucose management. Clinically significant hypoglycemia, as defined by the International Hypoglycemia Study Group, is a glucose level less than 54 mg/dL detected by CGM or SMBG. Severe hypoglycemia involves cognitive impairment severe enough to require the assistance of another person for recovery.[16] Patients should be counseled to alert their close contacts of the symptoms of hypoglycemia which can include shakiness, irritability, confusion, tachycardia, and hunger, among others. Severe and untreated hypoglycemia can progress to loss of consciousness, coma, and death.[4]

The ADA recommends that treatment of hypoglycemia be initiated at or less than the glucose alert value of 70 mg/dL. Treatment of conscious and cooperative patients typically consists of glucose containing food or tablets with 15 to 20 g of glucose every 15 minutes until the blood glucose level returns to normal. If the hypoglycemic person is unconscious or not willing to take oral glucose, a glucagon injection kit should be administered by whoever is in close contact with the patient, regardless of whether that person is a medical professional.[17]

Nutritional Management

The ADA applies the general diabetes nutrition principles to patients with type 1 or type 2 diabetes. The current recommendation includes a focus on healthy food patterns rather than strict diets. Foods that are nutrient dense and high quality are recommended, such as whole grains, fruits, vegetables, low-fat dairy, and lean proteins. Highly processed foods with added sugar are discouraged. The ADA also recommends an individualized medical nutrition therapy program provided by a registered dietician.[4] These interventions have been shown to decrease hemoglobin A1c values by nearly 1% in type 1 diabetics, particularly when carbohydrate counting is a primary focus.[18]

Patients who ask regarding nutritional supplements should be advised that without evidence of underlying deficiency, no benefit has been seen from additional herbal or nonherbal supplementation, such as cinnamon.[19]

Type 1 diabetic patients who consume alcohol are at increased risk for hypoglycemia in addition to traditional concerns regarding liver disease, cancer, cardiovascular, and safety concerns. Patients should be counseled to limit their alcohol consumption to 1 serving per day for women and 2 servings per day for men if consumed.[20] Type 1 diabetics should be counseled to consume food at the same time as alcohol to minimize the risk for delayed hypoglycemia, which can last up to 24 hours after alcohol consumption.[21]

Physical Activity

Physical activity has been well established to provide specific health benefits to the type 2 diabetes population; however, the benefit in type 1 diabetics is less clear and complicated by the danger of both hyperglycemia and hypoglycemia. A literature review conducted in 2015 concluded that statistical benefit related to exercise in type 1 diabetes was observed in the areas of physical fitness, strength, cardiovascular health, and well-being. However, no benefit, or unclear benefit, was described with regard to reduction of hemoglobin A1c.[22]

In general, adults with type 1 diabetes should be counseled to perform at least 150 minutes of moderate to intense exercise every week, divided over at least 3 days in addition to 2 to 3 resistance training sessions per week.[4] These general recommendations should be adjusted based on each patient's situation. Glucose should be assessed before exercise, and the ADA recommends that most patients should have a glucose level of 100 mg/dL or higher before initiating exercise.[1] Type 1 diabetic patients should be counseled to monitor for hypoglycemia during, immediately after, and about 7 to 11 hours after exercising, as hypoglycemia may occur owing to a lowering of glucose, as muscles replenish glycogen stores.[23]

Prevention and Screening

Type 1 diabetics are at increased risk for complications as a result of elevated glucose levels. These complications are commonly divided into macrovascular and microvascular categories. These conditions should be monitored at baseline and during the duration of follow-up.

Macrovascular complications

Type 1 diabetics are at increased risk for cardiovascular disease, even in the absence of standard risk factors such as hypertension, hyperlipidemia, smoking, and family history. There are no specific guidelines for screening examinations in the absence of symptoms or concerning physical examination findings.[13]

Blood pressure should be measured at each follow-up visit and treatment considered for sustained blood pressure of greater than 140/90 or greater than 130/80 in patients with additional risk factors. Angiotensin-converting enzyme inhibitors or angiotensin receptor blockers are the first-line drug for treatment of hypertension in diabetic patients.[4]

Lipids should be measured at diagnosis and annually along with assessment of weight and smoking status. The low-density lipoprotein goal for diabetic patients without atherosclerotic cardiovascular disease (ASCVD) is less than100 mg/dL and less than 70 mg/dL for those with ASCVD.[13] Moderate-intensity stain therapy is recommended for patients with diabetes age 40 to 75 and for patients younger than 40 with additional risk factors. Patients with existing ASCVD should be treated with high-intensity statins. Aspirin therapy is recommended as secondary prevention in diabetic patients with a history of ASCVD.[4]

Microvascular complications

Three main microvascular complications are neuropathy, nephropathy and retinopathy. These complications should be screened for at the initial evaluation and during follow up visits, and appropriate referrals made when indicated. Patients should be aware of the potential of these complications and notify providers of signs and symptoms.

Diabetic neuropathy is the most common microvascular complication observed in patients with longstanding diabetes. Many studies found that at least one-third of patients 40 years and older have neuropathy. Clinicians should perform a comprehensive foot examination on initial evaluation and then annually, including evaluation of the dorsalis pedis and posterior tibialis pulses; assessment of the patellar and Achilles reflexes; determination of proprioception, vibration, and monofilament sensation; and visual inspection.[13]

The risk of diabetic kidney disease is up to 50% in type 1 and type 2 diabetics. The primary prevention is glycemic control, and risk factors include long diabetes duration, hypertension, obesity, and smoking. Microalbuminuria is a marker and screening tool to detect diabetic kidney disease and should be evaluated along with serum creatinine at initial evaluation and annually thereafter.[13]

Diabetic retinopathy and its many forms are the most common cause of new cases of legal blindness.[13] In type 1 diabetes, most patients will have at least one form of diabetic retinopathy at 20 years' duration of disease, although fortunately, only 5% to 8% of type 1 diabetic patients have the more sight-threatening variations. Laser therapy does reduce the risk of blindness caused by diabetic retinopathy, and the screening examinations are aimed at identifying disease at detectable levels. Type 1 diabetic patients should be referred for expert diabetic retinal evaluation starting 5 years after diagnosis or earlier in the presence of symptoms or for unknown duration of diabetes. Examinations should continue annually in most cases.[13]

Other considerations

Patients with autoimmune-related diabetes are at risk for other autoimmune disease. Clinicians should consider screening for these disorders at the initial visit and thereafter based on the clinical findings and symptoms. Descriptions of the most common autoimmune disease seen in patients with type 2 diabetes are listed in **Fig. 3.**[4]

Age-specific hip fracture risk in patients with type 1 diabetes is increased to a relative risk of 6.3 compared with the general populations, regardless of gender.[4] Despite this risk, the recommendations for osteoporosis screening are the same as those for the general public. The current recommendation from the US Preventative Services Task Force is for baseline bone density examination for women age 65 and older and younger women with additional risk factors.[24]

Patients with diabetes are at increased risk for hospitalization from the flu, at increased risk for bacterial pneumonia, and are found to have higher rates of hepatitis B when compared with the general public; therefore, the ADA recommends that patients with type 1 diabetes receive the following vaccinations[4]:

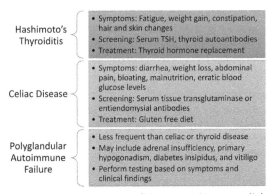

Hashimoto's Thyroiditis
- Symptoms: Fatigue, weight gain, constipation, hair and skin changes
- Screening: Serum TSH, thyroid autoantibodies
- Treatment: Thyroid hormone replacement

Celiac Disease
- Symptoms: diarrhea, weight loss, abdominal pain, bloating, malnutrition, erratic blood glucose levels
- Screening: Serum tissue transglutaminase or entiendomysial antibodies
- Treatment: Gluten free diet

Polyglandular Autoimmune Failure
- Less frequent than celiac or thyroid disease
- May include adrenal insufficiency, primary hypogonadism, diabetes insipidus, and vitiligo
- Perform testing based on symptoms and clinical findings

Fig. 3. Common co-existing autoimmune conditions seen in type 1 diabetes.

- Age-specific recommended vaccinations just as the regular population
- Annual flu vaccinations for diabetes ≥ 6 months
- Pneumococcal polysaccharide vaccine for patients 2 years or older
- Hepatitis B vaccination series for diabetics aged 19 to 59

Diabetes Education and Support

Just as living with type 1 diabetes is a continuous process, so should be diabetes education and support. All newly diagnosed diabetics should participate in diabetes self-management education (DSME) and diabetes self-management support (DSMS) to begin the process of buildings the knowledge, skills and behaviors necessary to live well with diabetes. Ongoing DSME and DSMS programs should also be offered annually, upon transition of care, and as needed to address patient specific changes in food and activity level, as well as social issues. These programs should support the patient and family in making informed decisions to improve their health status and quality of life.[1]

Research focused on the benefits of DSME have shown improvement in clinical data such as hemoglobin A1c, body weight, health care costs as well as patient reported improvements in quality of life and coping.[4] Unfortunately, participation rates for these programs are low, indicating that only 5% to 7% of eligible patients are completing DSME.[25] Reimbursable programs are traditionally limited to in person settings. The development of distance programs may improve patient participation, however, reimbursement from insurance plans is a barrier.

LONG-TERM OUTCOMES

Type 1 diabetes is associated with increased mortality, primarily related to the vascular consequences of the disease. The Pittsburgh Epidemiology of Diabetes Complications study showed that type 1 diabetic patients diagnosed in childhood and re-evaluated at age younger than 45 had an increased all-cause mortality of 5 times that of the age-matched general population. Cardiovascular disease mortality increased 20- to 30-fold, and for all outcomes, the risk to women was higher than in men.[26] Although it is thought that these statistics are improving in countries that spend more on health care,[27] clinicians and patients must continue to strive to control blood glucose and minimize long-term complications.

SUMMARY

Knowledge of the risk factors involved in the development of type 1 diabetes is continuing to evolve and stimulate research focused on early identification of individuals at risk for type 1 diabetes, preventing or halting the progression of disease, and curing patients already living with type 1 diabetes. Practitioners must be aware of current management goals and work with patients to provide ongoing motivation and education so that patients can minimize their risk for complications of type 1 diabetes. The hospitalized type 1 diabetic patient is at particular risk for poor outcomes, and clinicians should be vigilant to provide appropriate care. Long-term outcomes for patients with type 1 diabetes are improving, and clinicians should be aware of the potential complications from diabetes to help their patients live longer, healthier lives.

REFERENCES

1. Chiang JL, Kirkman MS, Laffel LM, et al. Type 1 diabetes through the life span: a position statement of the American Diabetes Association. Diabetes Care 2014;37(7):2034–54.

2. Centers for Disease Control and Prevention. National diabetes statistics report: estimates of diabetes and its burden in the United States, 2014. Atlanta (GA): US Department of Health and Human Services; 2014.

3. Forlenza GP, Rewers M. The epidemic of type 1 diabetes: what is it telling us? Curr Opin Endocrinol Diabetes Obes 2011;18(4):248–51.

4. American Diabetes Association. Standards of medical care in diabetes—2017 abridged for primary care providers. Clin Diabetes 2017;35(1):5–26.

5. Chae YK, Chiec L, Mohindra N, et al. A case of pembrolizumab-induced type-1 diabetes mellitus and discussion of immune checkpoint inhibitor-induced type 1 diabetes. Cancer Immunol Immunother 2017;66(1):25–32.

6. Ziegler AG, Rewers M, Simell O, et al. Seroconversion to multiple islet autoantibodies and risk of progression to diabetes in children. JAMA 2013;309(23): 2473–9.

7. Jovanovič L, Savas H, Mehta M, et al. Frequent monitoring of A1C during pregnancy as a treatment tool to guide therapy. Diabetes Care 2011;34(1):53–4.

8. Lee J-E. Alternative biomarkers for assessing glycemic control in diabetes: fructosamine, glycated albumin, and 1, 5-anhydroglucitol. Ann Pediatr Endocrinol Metab 2015;20(2):74–8.

9. Diabetes Control Complications Trial Research Group, Nathan DM, Genuth S, Lachin J, et al. The effect of intensive treatment of diabetes on the development and progression of long-term complications in insulin-dependent diabetes mellitus. N Engl J Med 1993;(329):977–86.

10. Diabetes Control Complications Trial Epidemiology of Diabetes Interventions Complications Research Group, Lachin JM, Genuth S, Cleary P, et al. Retinopathy and nephropathy in patients with type 1 diabetes four years after a trial of intensive therapy. N Engl J Med 2000;(342):381–9.

11. U.S. Food and Drug Administration. Dexcom G5 mobile continuous glucose monitoring system - P120005/S041. 2016. Available at: https://www.fda.gov/medicaldevices/productsandmedicalprocedures/deviceapprovalsandclearances/recently-approveddevices/ucm533969.htm. Accessed April 30, 2017.

12. Juvenile Diabetes Research Foundation Continuous Glucose Monitoring Study Group. Continuous glucose monitoring and intensive treatment of type 1 diabetes. N Engl J Med 2008;(359):1464–76.

13. Peters AL, Laffel LM, Chiang JL. The American Diabetes Association/JDRF type 1 diabetes sourcebook. Arlington (VA): American Diabetes Association; 2013.

14. Afrezza(R) [package insert]. Danbury, CT: MannKind Corporation; 2016. Available at: https://afrezza.com/wp-content/uploads/2016/08/afrezza.pdf. Accessed May 6, 2017.

15. SymlinPen(R) [package insert]. Wilmington, DE: AstraZeneca Pharmaceuticals LP; 2015. Available at: https://www.azpicentral.com/symlin/pi_symlin.pdf#page=1. Accessed May 6, 2017.

16. Seaquist ER, Anderson J, Childs B, et al. Hypoglycemia and diabetes: a report of a workgroup of the American Diabetes Association and the Endocrine Society. Diabetes Care 2013;36(5):1384–95.

17. Aghazadeh Y, Nostro MC. Cell therapy for type 1 diabetes: current and future strategies. Curr Diab Rep 2017;17(6):37.

18. Scavone G, Manto A, Pitocco D, et al. Effect of carbohydrate counting and medical nutritional therapy on glycaemic control in type 1 diabetic subjects: a pilot study. Diabet Med 2010;27(4):477–9.

19. Evert AB, Boucher JL, Cypress M, et al. Nutrition therapy recommendations for the management of adults with diabetes. Diabetes Care 2013;36(11): 3821–42.
20. Mozaffarian D. Dietary and policy priorities for cardiovascular disease, diabetes, and obesity. Circulation 2016;133(2):187–225.
21. Richardson T, Weiss M, Thomas P, et al. Day after the night before. Diabetes Care 2005;28(7):1801–2.
22. Chimen M, Kennedy A, Nirantharakumar K, et al. What are the health benefits of physical activity in type 1 diabetes mellitus? A literature review. Diabetologia 2012;55(3):542–51.
23. McMahon SK, Ferreira LD, Ratnam N, et al. Glucose requirements to maintain euglycemia after moderate-intensity afternoon exercise in adolescents with type 1 diabetes are increased in a biphasic manner. J Clin Endocrinol Metab 2007;92(3):963–8.
24. Nelson HD, Haney EM, Dana T, et al. Screening for osteoporosis: an update for the US Preventive Services Task Force. Ann Intern Med 2010;153(2):99–111.
25. Strawbridge LM, Lloyd JT, Meadow A, et al. Use of Medicare's diabetes self-management training benefit. Health Educ Behav 2015;42(4):530–8.
26. Miller RG, Mahajan HD, Costacou T, et al. A contemporary estimate of total mortality and cardiovascular disease risk in young adults with type 1 diabetes: the Pittsburgh epidemiology of diabetes complications study. Diabetes Care 2016; 39(12):2296–303.
27. Morgan E, Cardwell CR, Black CJ, et al. Excess mortality in type 1 diabetes diagnosed in childhood and adolescence: a systematic review of population-based cohorts. Acta Diabetol 2015;52(4):801–7.

The How-To for Type 2

An Overview of Diagnosis and Management of Type 2 Diabetes Mellitus

Seliece Dodds, MSN, ACNS-BC, APRN, CDE

KEYWORDS

- Type 2 diabetes • Hyperglycemia • Hemoglobin A1C • Metformin
- Microvascular complications • Macrovascular complications • Individualized care

KEY POINTS

- Type 2 diabetes and its associated comorbidities and complications are a national and world health issue.
- Patients with type 2 diabetes can develop various complications, including microvascular issues such as nephropathy, retinopathy, and peripheral neuropathy, as well as macrovascular damage.
- Targets for glycemic control, as well as nonpharmacological and pharmacologic interventions, should be individualized based on patient-specific characteristics.

INTRODUCTION

Type 2 diabetes (T2DM) and its associated comorbidities and complications are a national and world health issue. According to the World Health Organization (WHO), an estimated 180 million adults had diabetes in 1980, which climbed to 422 million by 2014.[1] T2DM, which previously was considered an adult-onset disorder, is increasing among children, adolescents, and young adults.[2] Since 1980, age-standardized diabetes prevalence has at best been unimproved in every country, and in most countries, numbers have increased.[1] The projected worldwide prevalence of diabetes is anticipated to reach 642 million by 2040.[3] T2DM, characterized by insulin resistance and increased hepatic glucose output, accounts for most of these cases.[4,5]

When diabetes is not well managed, and hyperglycemia persists for prolonged periods of time, patients with T2DM can develop various complications, including both microvascular issues such as nephropathy, retinopathy, and peripheral neuropathy, as well as macrovascular damage (eg, cardiovascular disease).[4] These complications

Disclosure Statement: No disclosures to report.
Division of Internal Medicine, Department of Endocrine Neoplasia and Hormonal Disorders, MD Anderson Cancer Center, 1515 Holcombe Boulevard, Unit 1461, Houston, TX 77030, USA
E-mail address: srdodds@mdanderson.org

Nurs Clin N Am 52 (2017) 513–522
http://dx.doi.org/10.1016/j.cnur.2017.07.002   nursing.theclinics.com

and associated comorbidities account for a huge medical cost burden. The full economic impact is considered difficult to estimate given its multifactorial nature, which includes both direct medical costs in addition to intangible factors such as a reduction quality of life due to stress, anxiety, and other psychosocial sequelae. Direct medical costs alone were estimated to total at least $129 million worldwide in 2003 for people aged 20 to 79 years.[4] The World Health Organization (WHO) estimated that in 2001, nearly 960,000 deaths worldwide were caused by diabetes, accounting for approximately 3% of all deaths caused by noncommunicable diseases.[4] In order to prevent diabetes-related complications, costs, and deaths, glycemic control measures have consistently been part of national and international diabetes and endocrinology guidelines. For example, the 2016 Consensus Statement by the American Association of Clinical Endocrinologists (AACE) lists hemoglobin A1C (A1C) targets and self-monitoring of blood glucose (SMBG) as foundational principles for T2DM management.[6] Because of the variety of socioeconomic, cultural, and age groups affected by the disease, guidelines advise a holistic patient-centered approach to care.[6] Additionally, guidelines encourage comprehensive medical evaluation and management of comorbidities. According to the American Diabetes Association (ADA), comorbidity evaluation should include, but is not limited to, cardiovascular disease, microvascular disease, foot care, obesity management, and various psychosocial factors.[7]

DIAGNOSIS OF TYPE 2 DIABETES

To understand recommended management of an illness, diagnostic criteria should first be addressed. The diagnosis of T2DM, according to the 1997 criteria of the ADA, include a fasting plasma glucose (FPG) value greater than or equal to 126 mg per deciliter (7.0 mmol/L), or plasma glucose value greater than or equal to 200 mg per deciliter (11.1 mmol/L) 2 hours after 75 g oral glucose load (2hPG).[8] A random plasma glucose of greater than or equal to 200 mg per deciliter in a patient with classic symptoms of hyperglycemia is also considered diagnostic.[9] Lastly, a hemoglobin A1C greater than or equal to 6.5% is defined as diagnostic when standardization is validated. A1C testing has become a widely used marker of more chronic hyperglycemia, as it reflects a 2- to 3-month average of blood glucose levels.[9] Although the test initially lacked standardization, the assays have now improved, and the International Expert Committee in 2008 endorsed A1C use for the diagnosis of diabetes.[10] FPG, 2hPG, and A1C criteria were redefined in 1997 by the Expert Committee on the Diagnosis and Classification of Diabetes Mellitus based on epidemiologic studies that evaluated the association between glucose values and the presence of retinopathy. The committee observed that retinopathy increased in a linear fashion above the glycemic thresholds noted here.[10] The choice of which test to employ is at times debated. Some argue that A1C has several advantages to testing plasma glucose levels, as it does not require fasting or have as strong a potential to be skewed by day-to-day variations affected by stress or illness.[9] However, A1C can misleading in certain groups such as those with certain hemoglobinopathies or anemia that can affect red blood cell turnover.[9] **Table 1** defines these criteria for the diagnosis of diabetes.

Although these criteria outline diagnosis of diabetes, they do not clarify etiology. Determining etiology often depends on the history of present illness and presenting circumstances. At diagnosis, a practitioner's evaluation should consider variables such as pancreatitis, use of exogenous steroids, pregnancy, ketonuria, and family history of type 1 diabetes in order to determine if additional testing is needed to establish etiology. If type 1 diabetes or other cause for beta (β)-cell destruction is anticipated, then plasma C-peptide level and markers of immune destruction such as

Table 1
Diabetes diagnostic criteria[a]

Diagnostic Test	Laboratory Result	Other Details
Hemoglobin A1C	Greater than or equal to 6.5%	A1C testing should be performed by a National Glycohemoglobin Standardization Program (NGSP)-certified method and Diabetes Control and Complication Trial_(DCCT)- standardized assay
Fasting Plasma Glucose	Greater than or equal to 126 mg/dL or 7.0 mmol/L	Fasting is defined as no caloric intake for at least 8 h prior
2-hour Plasma Glucose	Greater than or equal to 200 mg/dL or 11.1 mmol/L	Testing should be performed as defined by WHO, using a glucose load equivalent to 75 g of anhydrous glucose in water
Random Plasma Glucose	Greater than or equal to 200 mg/dL or 11.1 mmol/L	This diagnosis is only held for patients with classic symptoms of hyperglycemia[b] or hyperglycemic crisis[c]

[a] According to the 2011 American Diabetes Association Position Statement.[9]
[b] Symptoms of hyperglycemia are defined in this ADA statement as weight loss, polydipsia, polyuria, and blurred vision.
[c] Hyperglycemic crises are defined in this ADA statement as hyperglycemia with ketoacidosis or the nonketotic hyperosmolar syndrome.
Data from American Diabetes Association. Diagnosis and classification of diabetes mellitus. Diabetes Care 2011;34 Suppl 1:S62–9.

autoantibodies to glutamate decarboxylase (GAD65) should be considered.[9] Ultimately, the decision about which tests to use to confirm the diagnosis and clarify etiology are at the discretion of the health care professional, and repeat testing is often encouraged to confirm testing accuracy.[9]

GOALS OF TYPE 2 DIABETES MANAGEMENT

Once the diagnosis is established, the aforementioned laboratory testing and likely SMBG values remain important markers to monitor for glycemic control. The 2016 Consensus Statement by AACE encourages glycemic targets be individualized based on various factors, including life expectancy, age, hypoglycemia risk, comorbid conditions, duration of diabetes, patient motivation, and adherence.[6] The statement continues by encouraging that therapy, whether lifestyle and/or pharmacologic in nature, should be evaluated frequently (at least quarterly) until stable targets are achieved. When using A1C as a target, a range of less than 7% is often appropriate and can be safely achieved; however, in patients with advanced late-stage comorbidities or of very old age, tight control risks may outweigh benefits, and a goal an A1C goal closer to 8% may be considered reasonable.[11]

Regarding the factors of patient motivation and adherence, the environmental impact of resources and support system, as well as provider communication techniques, should be considered. When patient resources and support are readily available, more stringent glycemic targets may be advisable than when these elements are limited.[12] Decision making when possible should be made in conjunction with the patient and family, taking into account their preferences, values, and needs. In order to foster this collaboration, communication has been shown to be highly important. A recently published study by Polonsky and colleagues[13] evaluated physician-patient communication with patients at the diagnosis of T2DM and its links to patient outcomes. From November 2013 until January 2015, nearly 3700 people with T2DM from 26 countries were surveyed to evaluate 2 key components in care: (1) the diagnosis conversation, and (2) the conservation when additional oral medication was advised. The study reported that "patients' impressions of the quality of their communication with their physician at the diagnosis of T2DM are linked to their current well-being and self-care behavior." The discussion went on to highlight that encouragement as well as collaboration efforts were of particular value. With the diagnostic criteria, glycemic targets, as well as the emphasis of patient-centered care and collaboration in mind, the discussion should now progress toward management recommendations.

NONPHARMACOLOGICAL MANAGEMENT

Lifestyle optimization is essential for all patients with T2DM and is directed at modifiable risk factors, including body weight, physical activity, diet, sleep habits, psychosocial support, and tobacco use.[2,6] The ADA considers diet and exercise as first-line therapy in treatment of patients with T2DM.[5] Depending on the patient and his or her glycemic target, lifestyle modification may be the sole therapy or in addition to pharmacologic measures.[6] Diet counseling is often done on a focused referral to registered dietician, medical nutrition therapy counselor, and/or certified diabetes educator. The impact of dietary carbohydrates, especially refined sugars and processed foods, is a key factor to address. Additionally, the potential benefits of a plant-based diet with limited intake of saturated fatty acids and avoidance of transfats are considered key measures in some guidelines.[6] Foods high in fiber, including fruits, vegetables, legumes, and whole grains are encouraged in replacement of overly processed foods.[12] The newest ADA guidelines also encourage fat and protein counting in addition to carbohydrate counting for some patients.[7] For overweight or obese individuals, the goal of diet and exercise counseling is directed at safe, goal-oriented weight loss. These measures are focused on restriction of caloric intake and moderate physical activity for at least 150 minutes per week.[4] Five percent to 10% weight loss from baseline is advisable as a starting goal.[6] In addition to diet and exercise measures for weight loss, optimizing lifestyle is important for a nutritional deficiency perspective. For example, the most recent ADA guidelines recommend monitoring of vitamin B12 levels and potential supplementation in patients with long-term metformin use.[7] The addition of other vitamin supplements to a healthy diet is not generally recommended overall, as there is no clear evidence overall to support use outside of known deficiencies.[14] ADA Standards of Care have recently incorporated the recommendation to evaluate for diabetes comorbidities with assessment including, but not limited to, sleep disturbance, autoimmune disease, anxiety disorders, depression, and disordered eating.[7] Each of these have been associated with worsening diabetes management. Evidence supports that sleep deprivation has been associated with aggravating insulin resistance, hypertension, increased inflammatory cytokines, and dyslipidemia.[6]

Various research studies confirm the beneficial effects of lifestyle modification. For example, a multicenter, randomized clinical trial by the Diabetes Prevention Program Research Group published in the *New England Journal of Medicine* in 2002 demonstrated benefits of preventing T2DM progression in adults who were at high risk.[15] Over 3000 adults were randomized to placebo, metformin medication, or an intensive lifestyle-modification group. The goals in the lifestyle-modification group were at least 7% weight loss through a healthy, low-calorie, low-fat diet and to engage in at least 150 minutes of moderate-intensity physical activity per week. Those in the lifestyle-intervention group also received systematic and individualized counseling. All participants were followed for an average of 2.8 years, and 92.5% maintained follow up within 5 months of study closure. The cumulative incidence of diabetes was 31% and 58% lower in the metformin and lifestyle-modification groups respectively compared with placebo. The results were similar in men, women, racial and ethnic groups, as well as age groups. Metformin was shown to be less effective in persons with a lower baseline body mass index or a lower fasting plasma glucose concentration compared with those with a higher baseline. The reduction in fasting plasma glucose levels was similar in metformin and lifestyle groups, but the reduction in glycosylated hemoglobin levels was greater in the lifestyle intervention group. The summary estimates that lifestyle intervention as employed in the study can be estimated to prevent 1 case of T2DM per 7 persons who follow the measures for 3 years.[15]

PHARMACOLOGIC MANAGEMENT OF HYPERGLYCEMIA

When lifestyle modifications are not adequate to bring a patient to personalized glucose target, medications should be considered to supplement these measures. As discussed previously, a one-size-fits-all approach to glycemic management is no longer recommended; rather personalization based on patient characteristics is advised.[16] For patients with an A1C less than 7%, diet and exercise alone may be adequate unless symptomatology and/or plans for pregnancy or other rationale for tighter control be necessitated.[5] However, less stringent targets may be considered for some patient groups such as the elderly and/or those with poor health status or complex comorbidities.[16] When diet and exercise measures are deemed inadequate, monotherapy with metformin, unless contraindicated, is most often the first consideration, along with close monitoring to assess for improvement and evaluation of the need for changed or additional pharmacotherapy thereafter.[5] However, for patients with an A1C above 9% or for those with symptomatic hyperglycemia, initiating treatment with combination therapy is advised at least temporarily to relieve glucose toxicity.[11] Regarding metformin contraindication, it should be noted that recent US Food and Drug Administration (FDA) recommendations extended metformin's use to include patients with mild-moderate, stable chronic kidney disease with contraindication set at an estimated glomerular filtration rate (GFR) of less than 30 mL/min/1.73 m^2.[16] A strong consensus for metformin monotherapy revolves around its longstanding safety record, high efficacy, low cost, weight neutrality, and reasonable tolerability.[3,6,11] In cases where metformin is contraindicated, nonpreferred due to patient characteristics, or its use does not bring a patient to glycemic target, there are numerous options for an additional or alternative agent. All FDA-approved medications for the treatment of T2DM lower A1C by 0.6% to 1.5%.[3] Currently, there are 10 classes of noninsulin, FDA approved antihyperglycemic agents in addition to the biguanide, metformin.[11,17] These classes include the following

- Insulin secretagogue sulfonylureas
- Alpha-glucosidase inhibitors
- Glinides
- Amylin analogue pramlintide
- Glucagon-like peptide 1 receptor agonists (GLP-1 RA)
- Dipeptidyl peptidase-4 inhibitors (DPP4i)
- Bile acid sequestrant colesevelam

- Dopamine-2 agonist bromocriptine
- Thiazolidinediones
- Sodium glucose transporter 2 inhibition agents (SGLT-2i)

The choice of diabetes medication should take into consideration efficacy, mechanism of action, risk of hypoglycemia, tolerability, ease of use or administration, cost, risk of weight changes, and safety with comorbid conditions.[6] When adding a medication, a practitioner should consider its interactions with other diabetes medications and aim to prescribe agents that may work in a complementary fashion. Guidelines from the ADA indicate that any of these FDA-approved second agents can be used in combination with metformin. The AACE, on the other hand, advises considering either SGLT-2i or incretin-based therapies (GLP-1 RA or DPP4i).[3]

When a patient is unable to reach target with these pharmacologic options, whether because of nonefficacy, contraindication, cost burden, or adverse effect profile, insulin should be considered for management. Insulin is considered the most potent glucose-lowering agent.[6] Thus, the addition of basal with or without prandial insulin should be made cautiously and determined based on SMBG trends and patient-specific targets.[3] The 2016 AACE consensus recommends that insulin should be considered when patients have an A1c above 8% while taking 2 non-insulin anti-hyperglycemic agents and/or have long-standing diabetes and are unlikely to reach personalized A1C target with a third noninsulin agent.[6]

MANAGEMENT OF DIABETES-ASSOCIATED COMORBIDITIES

Management of diabetes should be holistic and, thus, incorporate monitoring and treatment of disease-related comorbidities. Intervening with lifestyle changes and potentially pharmacologic treatment to assist with glycemic control as discussed are primary measures for prevention. However, additional efforts may be necessarily employed for adequate prevention and detection. Both microvascular and macrovascular complications should be addressed.

Microvascular complications include nephropathy, retinopathy, and neuropathy. Nephropathy, or kidney disease, should be screened with at least an annual test of urine albumin excretion in patients with T2DM starting at diagnosis.[18] Additionally, estimated GFR should be evaluated and if less than 60 mL/min/1.73 m^2, chronic kidney disease and its management should be considered.[18] Optimizing both blood glucose and blood pressure control are essential for reducing the risk and slowing the progression of nephropathy. Referral to a nephrologist may be advisable. Blood glucose control, blood pressure management, and consultation among health care providers are also necessitated in the evaluation of another microvascular complication, retinopathy. The ADA recommends that patients with T2DM should have an initial comprehensive eye examination with dilation shortly after diagnosis.[18] Follow-up eye examination with high-quality fundus photographs alongside a comprehensive eye examination is recommended annually. For patients with known complications such as macular edema, severe nonproliferative diabetic retinopathy (NPDR), or any proliferative diabetic retinopathy (PDR), closer monitoring and treatment should be advised. Therapy with laser photocoagulation is indicated to reduce vision loss risk in patients with high-risk PDR and some cases of NPDR. For diabetic macular edema, antivascular endothelial growth factor (VEGF) therapy is indicated. The intervals of monitoring and selection of treatment should be made in collaboration with a trained eye care provider.[18] Finally, regarding microvascular complications, peripheral neuropathy should be addressed in a timely and coordinated manner. The most common symptoms of neuropathy are numbness, tingling, and pain in the feet and potentially hands, that is worse at rest and tends to improve with movement. Screening for distal symmetric polyneuropathy is recommended to start at diagnosis of T2DM and at least annually thereafter.[18] In conjunction with review of systems to assess for neuropathy systems, a physical examination specifically of the feet is indicated. Foot examination should include inspection of skin integrity, toenails, and foot deformities, as well as assessment of posterior tibial and dorsalis pedis pulses and for sensation. Testing for loss of protective sensation (LOPS) can be done using the 10 g monofilament plus vibration with a 128 Hz tuning fork, ankle reflexes, or pin prink sensation.[18] Additional foot evaluation may include ankle-brachial index for patients with suspected peripheral arterial disease. Management for all patients should begin with education of general foot self-care measures. However, as with all microvascular complications, a collaborative and multidisciplinary approach is recommended, especially for patients at high risk as referrals to podiatry and/or nerve specialists may be advisable.[18]

Concerning macrovascular disease, atherosclerosis is highly prevalent in patients with T2DM, and management to reduce risk or prevent coronary artery disease (CAD) is of high importance.[12] In asymptomatic patients, routine screening of CAD is not recommended, but those with known cardiovascular disease should have close monitoring and treatment.[18] in regards to CAD risk factors, monitoring and management of hypertension and hyperlipidemia is fundamental. Patients with T2DM who also have elevated blood pressure are at increased risk for cardiovascular events compared with diabetes without hypertension.[6] AACE recommends, as with A1C targets, that blood pressure goals be individualized, noting, however, that a target of less than 130 over 80 mm Hg is appropriate for most patients. The ADA sets its blood pressure target based on a systolic blood pressure goal of less than 140 mm Hg; however, the 2014 guideline notes that systolic blood pressure less than 130 may be appropriate for certain individuals.[18] To help patients reach this blood pressure target, therapy may consist of weight loss, sodium restriction, moderating alcohol intake, exercise, and pharmacologic treatment. If a patient requires pharmacologic management to reach the goal, angiotensin-converting enzyme inhibitors (ACEis) or angiotensin II receptor blockers (ARBs) have been considered optimal, as these classes have also been shown to slow progression of nephropathy and retinopathy.[6] For patients without albuminuria, thiazide-like diuretics and dihydropyridine calcium channel blockers should be considered due to the known beneficial cardiovascular outcomes.[7] Similar to hypertension, hyperlipidemia has a marked impact on comorbidity status. High cholesterol increases one's risk of arteriosclerotic cardiovascular disease, and in patients with T2DM, that risk is increased.[19] Stratifying patients based on their risk of ASCVD can help guide clinicians in management. Low-density lipoprotein (LDL-C) measurements currently serve as the target measure. For patients considered high risk or very high risk, goals of LDL-C less than 100 mg/dL or less than 70 mg/dL are respectively advised.[6] Many patients with T2DM can achieve lipid target(s) with lifestyle therapy, including healthy diet, physical activity, weight loss, and smoking cessation. However, for those who do not reach LDL goal, the AACE advises that the first-line pharmacologic treatment should be statin, unless contraindicated.[6] Lipid panels are advised to be evaluated at least every 2 years.[18]

SUMMARY

T2DM undoubtedly has widespread impact. The burden of the disease is widespread, with an impact on global costs, rise in epidemiologic comorbidities, risk of increased mortality, and decline in individuals' quality-of-life. These impact the practitioner's

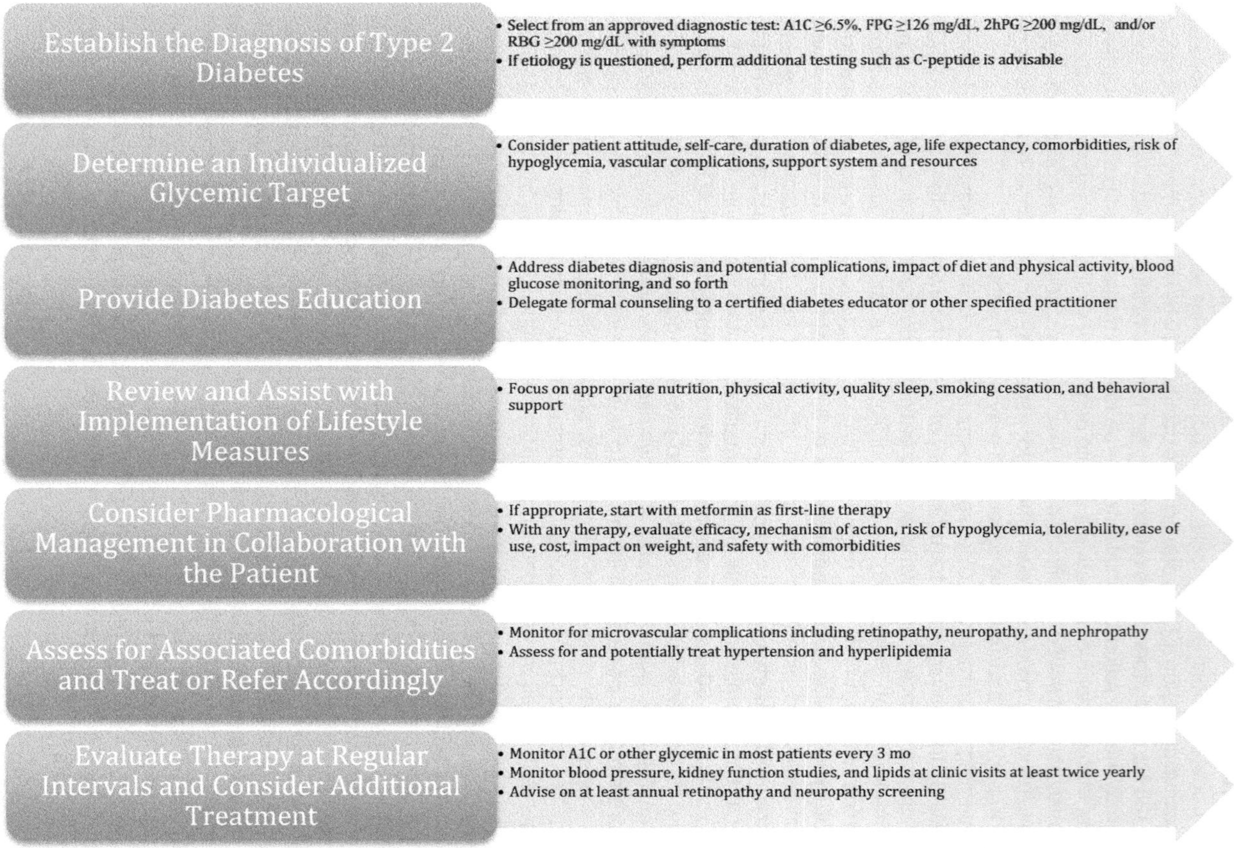

Fig. 1. Potential step-wise approach to type 2 diabetes management.

management of patients due to personalized effects. A step-wise approach is often recommended to help ease these burdens.

The multifactorial impact of T2DM on various organ systems may provide 1 approach to management. Knowledge of the disease has expanded markedly over the past decade. The pathophysiology of diabetes was described in 1988 by DeFronzo as the "terrible triumvirate," which highlighted 3 aspects of the disease: impaired insulin secretion, decreased peripheral glucose uptake, and increased hepatic glucose production.[11,20] However, over the 20 years following, the pathologic effects T2DM expanded to include various other abnormalities. In 2009, DeFronzo published an article in *Diabetes,* called "From the Triumvirate to the Ominous Octet: A New Paradigm for the Treatment of Type 2 Diabetes Mellitus." The "ominous octet" expounded upon the previous model and was illustrated to include renal glucose excretion changes, neurotransmitter dysfunction, increased lipolysis, increased glucose reabsorption from the gut, and increased hepatic glucagon production.[11,20] The goal of this model was to provide an "alternate therapeutic algorithm" that was based upon pathophysiologic changes in T2DM rather than on reduction in plasma glucose concentrations alone.[20]

Fazel outlined another method to help practitioners determine treatment.[16] This method was adapted to incorporate additional data from the 2016 AACE consensus statement[6] and is illustrated in Diagram 1. Ultimately, an evidence-based, patient-centered approach to patient care is fundamental in achieving sustainable and impactful management of T2DM. Further emphasis on prevention will be critical to reducing the widespread incidence of T2DM, particularly in younger populations **Fig. 1.**

REFERENCES

1. Collaboration NRF. Worldwide trends in diabetes since 1980: a pooled analysis of 751 population-based studies with 4.4 million participants. Lancet 2016; 387(10027):1513–30.
2. Chen L, Magliano DJ, Zimmet PZ. The worldwide epidemiology of type 2 diabetes mellitus–present and future perspectives. Nat Rev Endocrinol 2011;8(4): 228–36.
3. Reusch JE, Manson JE. Management of type 2 diabetes in 2017: getting to goal. JAMA 2017;317(10):1015–6.
4. Venkat Narayan KM, Zhang P, Kanaya AM, et al. Diabetes: the pandemic and potential solutions. Disease Control Priorities in Developing Countries 2006;2: 591–603. Available at: https://www.ncbi.nlm.nih.gov/pubmed/21250351.
5. Luna B, Feinglos MN. Oral agents in the management of type 2 diabetes mellitus. Am Fam Physician 2001;63(9):1747–56.
6. Garber AJ, Abrahamson MJ, Barzilay JI, et al. Consensus Statement by the American Association of Clinical Endocrinologists and American College of Endocrinology on the comprehensive type 2 diabetes management algorithm–2016 executive summary. Endocr Pract 2016;22(1):84–113.
7. Standards of medical care in diabetes-2017: summary of revisions. Diabetes Care 2017;40(Suppl 1):S4–5.
8. Gavin JR, Alberti K, Davidson MB, et al. Report of the expert committee on the diagnosis and classification of diabetes mellitus. Diabetes Care 1997;20(7): 1183–97.
9. American Diabetes Association. Diagnosis and classification of diabetes mellitus. Diabetes Care 2011;34(Suppl 1):S62–9.

10. Committee IE. International Expert Committee report on the role of the A1C assay in the diagnosis of diabetes. Diabetes Care 2009;32(7):1327–34.
11. Cavaiola TS, Pettus JH. Management of type 2 diabetes: selecting amongst available pharmacological agents. In: De Groot LJ, Chrousos G, Dungan K, et al, editors. Endotext [Internet]. South Dartmouth (MA): MDText.com, Inc; 2000.
12. Inzucchi SE, Bergenstal RM, Buse JB, et al. Management of hyperglycemia in type 2 diabetes: a patient-centered approach. Diabetes Care 2012;35(6): 1364–79.
13. Polonsky WH, Capehorn M, Belton A, et al. Physician-patient communication at diagnosis of type 2 diabetes and its links to patient outcomes: new results from the global IntroDia(R) study. Diabetes Res Clin Pract 2017;127:265–74.
14. Yan MK, Khalil H. Vitamin supplements in type 2 diabetes mellitus management: a review. Diabetes Metab Syndr 2017. [Epub ahead of print].
15. Group DPPR. Reduction in the incidence of type 2 diabetes with lifestyle intervention or metformin. N Engl J Med 2002;346(6):393–403.
16. Fazel MT, Pendergrass ML. Individualizing treatment of hyperglycemia in type 2 diabetes. JCOM 2017;24(1):23–38.
17. Raz I, Riddle MC, Rosenstock J, et al. Personalized management of hyperglycemia in type 2 diabetes: reflections from a diabetes care editors' expert forum. Diabetes Care 2013;36(6):1779–88.
18. American Diabetes Association. Executive summary: standards of medical care in diabetes—2014. Diabetes Care 2014;37(Suppl 1):S5–13.
19. Thom T, Haase N, Rosamond W, et al. Heart disease and stroke statistics–2006 update: a report from the American Heart Association Statistics Committee and Stroke Statistics Subcommittee. Circulation 2006;113(6):e85.
20. DeFronzo RA. From the triumvirate to the ominous octet: a new paradigm for the treatment of type 2 diabetes mellitus. Diabetes 2009;58(4):773–95.

Noninsulin Diabetes Medications

Sigi Varghese, RN, MSN, FNP-C, BC-ADM

KEYWORDS

- Diabetes medications • Alpha-glucosidase inhibitors • Biguanides • Meglitinides
- Dipeptidyl peptidase 4 inhibitors • Glucagon like peptide–1 agonists
- Selective sodium-glucose transporter-2 inhibitors • Sulfonylureas

KEY POINTS

- Type 2 diabetes can be treated with noninsulin diabetes medications using one drug alone or in combination with different drugs.
- Important properties of the antihyperglycemic agents play a role in the choice of that particular medication for individual patients.
- Selection of antidiabetic medications should be done carefully based on efficacy, impact on weight, hypoglycemia risk, potential side effects, cost, and patient preferences.

INTRODUCTION

The prevalence and incidence of type 2 diabetes (T2DM) are increasing worldwide. In the United States, 29.1 million people or 9.3% of population have diabetes,[1] of which 90% to 95% of people have T2DM. T2DM is the leading cause of cardiovascular disorders, blindness, kidney failure, and amputations. People with diabetes are hospitalized frequently and also have an increased risk of cancer,[2] mental illness,[3] cognitive decline,[4] liver disease,[5] and other disabling conditions. Effective management of diabetes is important to prevent and delay complications associated with diabetes.[1,6] Medical management of diabetes has become increasingly complex and several guidelines and recommendations have been developed to treat diabetes. Hemoglobin A1C target is the major focus of diabetes management.[6,7] The American Diabetes Association recommends lowering hemoglobin A1c to less than 7.0% in most patients to decrease the incidence of microvascular disease.[7]

Understanding the pathophysiology of diabetes is important to understand its management. Abnormal islet cell function is the key feature of T2DM. In the early stages of disease, insulin production is normal or can be increased, but insulin sensitivity is reduced. Pancreatic beta cells' ability to adequately produce insulin in the presence

Disclosure Statement: There are no commercial or financial conflicts of interest.
Department of Endocrine Neoplasia and Hormonal Disorders, The University of Texas MD Anderson Cancer Center, 1515 Holcombe Boulevard, Houston, Texas, 77030, USA
E-mail address: ssvarghese@mdanderson.org

of elevated glucose levels is compromised and this incompetence progresses over time. In T2DM, the pancreatic alpha cells secrete more glucagon, which promotes hepatic glucose output. Abnormalities in the incretion system glucagon like peptide-1 and glucose-dependent insulinotropic peptide causes hyperglycemia. Insulin resistance in the target tissues like liver, adipose tissue, and muscle causes hyperglycemia, especially in obese patients. An increased delivery of fatty acids to the liver and their oxidation contributes to increased gluconeogenesis.[8]

It is possible to reverse islet dysfunctions and improve hyperglycemia by enhancing the action of insulin, which decreases beta cell secretory burden. Restriction of dietary intake, bariatric surgery, and use of various antidiabetic medications can improve beta cell dysfunction. The antihyperglycemic agents are directed toward one or more of the above pathophysiologic defects. Many patients may need more than 1 class of medications to adequately treat diabetes.[7] Each medication's properties should be kept in mind when selecting a particular therapy for an individual patient.[6]

CLASSES OF NONINSULIN DIABETES MEDICATIONS

Pharmacologic therapy of T2DM now has changed greatly owing to new drugs and drug classes available. Noninsulin diabetes medications available in the United States to treat diabetes are as follows.

- Biguanide
- Sulfonylureas
- Meglitinide derivatives
- Alpha-glucosidase inhibitors
- Thiazolidinediones
- Glucagonlike peptide-1 (GLP-1) agonists
- Dipeptidyl peptidase 4 (DPP-4) Inhibitors
- Selective sodium glucose transporter - 2 (SGLT-2) inhibitors
- Amylinomimetic
- Bile acid sequestrant
- Dopamine agonist

Biguanide

This class is the first line treatment for T2DM and prediabetes and is the most widely prescribed diabetes medication. A biguanide decreases insulin resistance and improves insulin sensitivity, and this class is considered to be a cornerstone in the treatment of T2DM. Biguanide reduce hyperglycemia primarily by decreasing hepatic gluconeogenesis and secondarily by increasing the peripheral insulin sensitivity. Metformin does not increase insulin levels or cause weight gain or hypoglycemia, and it is effective, safe, and inexpensive. Metformin may reduce risk of cardiovascular events and death.[9,10] Metformin is administered orally as immediate release tablets, extended release tablets, or as an oral solution (**Table 1**).

Sulfonylureas

Sulfonylureas are insulin secreatagogues that stimulate the release of insulin from pancreatic beta cells, decrease the rate of hepatic glucose production, and increase insulin receptor sensitivity. It can reduce hemoglobin A1c by 1% to 2%; however, as beta cell dysfunction progresses, sulfonylureas become less effective.[11,12] The main advantage is that it is inexpensive. The main side effect is hypoglycemia. Glyburide, glipizide, and glimepiride are second-generation sulfonylureas

Table 1
Biguanide (Glucophage, Glucophage XR, Riomet, Fortamet, Glumetza)

Dosage forms and strengths	Immediate release tablets are available in 500, 850, and 1000 mg. Extended release tablets are available in 500, 750, and 1000 mg. Oral solution is available as 100 mg/mL.
Initiation and maintenance	Immediate release tablets or solution: start 500 mg twice daily or 850 mg/d with meals then increase every 2 wk. Continue as tolerated between 1500 and 2550 mg/d in divided doses every 8–12 h with meal, not to exceed 2550 mg/d. Extended-release tablets: Glucophage XR: Start 500 mg/d with dinner; titrate by 500 mg/d every week, not to exceed 2000 mg/d. Fortamet: Start 500–1000 mg/d, titrate by 500 mg/d every week; not to exceed 2500 mg/d. Glumetza: Start 1000 mg orally daily titrate by 500 mg/d every week, not to exceed 2000 mg/d.
Dosing modifications	In renal impairment: GFR <30 mL/min: contraindicated. GFR 30–45 mL/min: not recommended to initiate treatment. GFR falls below 45 mL/min while taking metformin, risks and benefits of continuing the therapy should be evaluated. Avoid use of metformin in hepatic impairment.
Pharmacology	Not metabolized by liver. It is rapidly eliminated unchanged by the kidneys. Drug levels increase markedly in renal insufficiency, which can lead to lactic acidosis. Half-life: 4–9 h.
Precautions	Discontinue before receiving IV contrast studies. Hold on the day of the procedure and reevaluate renal function 48 h after the procedure and restart if stable. Hold for surgery and procedures while the patient has restricted food and fluid intake. Avoid heavy alcohol use while on metformin. May cause vitamin B_{12} deficiency.[7] Check B_{12} levels annually.
Contraindications	Hypersensitivity, congestive heart failure, acute or chronic metabolic acidosis, diabetic ketoacidosis, GFR <30 mL/min.
Adverse reactions	Metallic taste in the mouth, anorexia, nausea, abdominal discomfort, and soft bowel movements or diarrhea.[9] To minimize side effects, metformin is usually taken with meals, and initiated at a low dose and increased as tolerated.
Pregnancy	Category B. Metformin enters breast milk so it is not recommended during lactation.

Abbreviations: GFR, glomerular filtration rate; IV, intravenous.

and are more potent with fewer drug interactions compared with first-generation sulfonylureas (**Table 2**).

Meglitinides

Meglitinides are shorter-acting insulin secretagogues than sulfonylureas. Meglitinides increase insulin secretion by binding to and closing the adenosine triphosphate-sensitive potassium channels. They are given before meals, which causes more physiologic release of insulin and less risk for hypoglycemia. The efficacy of meglitinide monotherapy is similar to that of sulfonylureas. Meglitinides are usually recommended if treatment with sulfonylurea fails or when postprandial hypoglycemia occurs with use

Table 2 Sulfonylureas	
Agent	**Comment**
Glyburide (Diabeta, Micronase)	
Dosage forms and strengths	Regular tablets available as 1.25, 2.5, and 5 mg. Micronized tablets available as 1.5, 3, 5, and 6 mg.
Initiation and maintenance	Start regular tab at 2.5–5 mg/d, maintain between 1.25 and 20 mg/d or twice daily but not to exceed 20 mg/d, consider administering twice daily for doses >10 mg/d. Start micronized tablets at 1.5–3 mg/d (patients at risk for hypoglycemia initiate at 0.75 mg/d), maintain at 0.75–12 mg/d, not to exceed 12 mg/d.
Pharmacology	Onset is within 15–60 min after a single dose, peak is 2–4 h, and duration is <24 h.
Glipizide (Glucotrol, Glucotrol XL)	
Dosage forms and strengths	Immediate release tablets available in 5 and 10 mg. Extended-release tablets available as 2.5, 5, and 10 mg.
Initiation and maintenance	Start immediate release tablets at 5 mg/d, increase by 2.5–5 mg as needed every several days. Maintain at 2.5–20 mg/d or every 12 h, not to exceed 40 mg/d. Initiate extended-release tablets (Glucotrol XL) at 5 mg/d given with breakfast; dose adjustment should not be done more frequently than every 7 d. Maintain 5–10 mg/d, not to exceed 20 mg/d.
Dosing modifications	Hepatic impairment: initiate 2.5 mg/d (immediate release). Renal impairment: If GFR is <50 mL/min, decrease dose by 50%.
Pharmacology	Onset is 30 min and max effect within 2–3 h. Duration of action 12–24 h. Half-life: 2–5 h (Glucotrol).
Glimepiride (Amaryl)	
Dosage forms and strengths	Available as 1-, 2-, and 4-mg tablets.
Initiation and maintenance	Initiate 1–2 mg orally in the morning after breakfast or with first meal; may increase dose by 1–2 mg every 1–2 wk; not to exceed 8 mg/d.
Dosing modifications	Renal impairment: 1 mg/d, titrate dose based on fasting blood glucose levels. Not recommended in severe hepatic impairment; initiate therapy with 1 mg/d and titrate carefully
Pharmacology	Initial effect within 1 h, duration of action 24 h, half-life 5–9 h.
Common issues in all sulfonylureas	
Precautions	Renal dysfunction, older patients, debilitated, malnourished, adrenal or pituitary insufficiency, infection, fever, trauma, or surgery, hepatic or renal insufficiency.
Contraindications	Hypersensitivity, sulfa allergy, type 1 diabetes, and diabetic ketoacidosis.
Adverse reactions	Hypoglycemia, hemolytic anemia can occur with glucose 6-phosphate dehydrogenase deficiency.
Pregnancy	Category C; not known if crosses into breast milk so avoid use in nursing women.

Abbreviation: GFR, glomerular filtration rate.

of sulfonylurea. Disadvantages of this therapy include the need for frequent dosing and cost[8,13] (**Table 3**).

Alpha-Glucosidase Inhibitors

Alpha-glucosidase inhibitors delay the digestion and absorption of carbohydrates and help to prevent postprandial hyperglycemia. They inhibit the upper gastrointestinal enzymes that convert complex polysaccharide carbohydrates into monosaccharides. Their effect on glycemic control is modest.[15,16] Alpha-glucosidase inhibitor's pharmacologic effects make it possible to use this therapy in the treatment of nondiabetic postprandial hypoglycemia that happens in patients with rapid gastric emptying, impaired glucose tolerance, and isolated reactive hypoglycemia.[15]

Table 3 Meglitinides	
Agent	**Comment**
Repaglinide (Prandin)[13]	
Dosage forms and strengths	0.5-, 1-, and 2-mg tablets.
Initiation and maintenance	Initiate 0.5 mg with no prior treatment and 1–2 mg with prior treatment. Can titrate up to 4 mg with meal but not to exceed 16 mg/d. Take dose 15 min before meal.
Dosing modifications	Renal impairment: CrCl 20–40 mL/min: 0.5 mg with meals; titrate slowly. CrCl <20 mL/min, no data available.
Pharmacology	Onset of action: 15–60 min, duration: 4–6 h. Half-life: 1 h.
Nateglinide	
Dosage forms and strengths	Available as 60 mg and 120 mg tablets.
Initiation and maintenance	Initiate 120 mg orally every 8 h, start 60 mg every 8 h if patient is near the hemoglobin A1c goal. Take dose 1–30 min before meal.
Pharmacology	Initial effect 15 min, duration of action 4 h, half-life 1.2–3 h.
Precautions all meglitinides	Coadministration of gemfibrozil results in an 8-fold increase in repaglinide plasma concentration, infection, trauma, fever and surgery, hepatic or renal insufficiency, patients who are elderly, debilitated, malnourished, and those with adrenal or pituitary insufficiency. Not indicated to use in combination with NPH insulin as myocardial ischemia has been reported.[14]
Common issues in all meglitinides	
Contraindications	Hypersensitivity, diabetic ketoacidosis, type I diabetes mellitus, use with other oral secretagogues.
Adverse reactions	Hypoglycemia, headache, and upper respiratory tract infection. Less common side effects are cardiovascular ischemia, diarrhea, constipation, urinary tract infection, hypersensitivity reactions, and sinusitis.
Pregnancy	Category: C, Not known if repaglinide crosses into breast milk so avoid use. Use of Nateglinide during lactation is unsafe.

Abbreviation: CrCl, creatinine kinase.

Available alpha-glucosidase inhibitors include acarbose, voglibose, and miglitol. They can be used as monotherapy or in combination with other treatment modalities. Alpha- glucosidase inhibitors may be less effective if eating low-carbohydrate meals (**Table 4**).

Thiazolidinediones

Thiazolidinediones are insulin-sensitizing agents that improve the target cell response and decrease hepatic gluconeogenesis. These agents reduce insulin resistance in the periphery by sensitizing skeletal muscle and adipose, and the liver to the actions of insulin.[17] The major action of thiazolidinediones is fat redistribution. These drugs also have beta cell preservation properties.[17] The US Food and Drug Administration–approved thiazolidinediones include pioglitazone and rosiglitazone. Both are indicated as an adjunct to diet and exercise to improve glycemic control in T2DM.[17] Because data suggested an elevated risk of myocardial infarction in patients treated with rosiglitazone, this agent is currently available only via a restricted access program. Because of cardiovascular safety concerns, rosiglitazone is not given to new patients unless they are unable to achieve glucose control on other medications and are not willing to take pioglitazone. The US Food and Drug Administration restricted access for rosiglitazone and combination products

Table 4 Alphaglucosidase inhibitors	
Agent	**Comment**
Acarbose (Precose)	
Dosage forms and strengths	Available as tablet 25, 50, and 100 mg.
Initiation and maintenance	Initially 25 mg orally 3 times a day with meals (with first bite). Can increase to 50 or 100 mg every 8 h at 4- to 8-wk intervals. Maximum dose: if <60 kg: 150 mg/d and if more than 60 kg 300 mg/d.
Dosing modifications	If creatinine is >2 avoid use. Contraindicated in liver cirrhosis.
Pharmacology	Half-life: 2 h.
Miglitol (Glyset)	
Dosage forms and strengths	Available as tablet, 25, 50, and 100 mg.
Initiation and maintenance	Start: 25 mg orally every 8 h at meals for 4–8 wk, then 50 mg every 8 h for 3 mo maximum 100 mg every 8 h.
Dosing modifications	Hepatic impairment: no adjustment necessary. Renal impairment: avoid use if creatinine >2.
Pharmacology	Half-life 2 h.
Common issues in all alphaglucosidase inhibitors	
Precautions	Creatinine >2, use glucose, not sucrose to treat hypoglycemia.
Contraindications	Ketoacidosis, cirrhosis, inflammatory bowel disease, colonic ulceration, partial or predisposition to intestinal obstruction, malabsorption, severe digestive disease.
Adverse reactions	Flatulence, diarrhea, and abdominal discomfort.
Pregnancy	Category B. It is not known if acarbose crosses into breast milk, avoid using in nursing women, miglitol enters slightly into breast milk so its use not recommended.

in September 2010 so they are not available in retail pharmacies.[17] Thiazolidine-diones cannot be used for acute management of hyperglycemia because it takes about 6 weeks to reach a steady state (**Table 5**).

Glucagonlike Peptide-1 Agonists

GLP-1 agonists lower blood sugar by stimulating glucose-dependent insulin release, reducing glucagon, and slowing gastric emptying. They release insulin based on high glucose levels as opposed to oral insulin secretagogues, which may cause non–glucose-dependent insulin release even in the presence of low blood sugar levels.[6,19] GLP-1 agonists help to promote weight loss.[20]

Table 5
Thiazoladinediones

Agent	Comment
Pioglitazone (Actos)	
Dosage forms and strengths	Available as15-, 30-, and 45-mg tablet.
Initiation and maintenance	Start 15–30 mg/d with meal, may increase dose by 15 mg to 45 mg/d maximum.
Dosing modifications	No renal dosage adjustment is needed. Pioglitazone should not be used if the ALT level is >2.5 times the upper limit of normal.
Pharmacology	Initial effect is delayed and maximum effect is after several weeks. Half-life: 3–7 h.
Rosiglitazone (Avandia)	
Dosage forms and strengths	Available as tablet: 2 and 4 mg.
Initiation and maintenance	Start 4 mg/d, or divided twice daily. If inadequate response after 8–12 wk, may increase dose to 8 mg/d or divided every 12 h.
Dosing modifications	Do not initiate rosiglitazone in active liver disease (ALT >2.5 times of upper limit normal. In renal impairment no dosage adjustments required.
Pharmacology	Onset of action: initial effect delayed; maximum effect may take up to 12 wk. Half-life: 3–4 h.
Common issues in thiazolidinediones	
Precautions	Can cause or exacerbate congestive heart failure in some at initiation as well as after dose increases, observe patients carefully for signs and symptoms of heart failure including excessive, rapid weight gain; dyspnea; and/or edema, congestive heart failure, New York Heart Class functional I and II, use with insulin, T1DM, DKA, baseline ALT >2.5 times the upper limit of normal, history of or active bladder cancer, hepatic impairment: monitor ALT at start of treatment, every month for 12 mo, then every 3 mo thereafter.
Contraindications	Black box warning: New York Heart Association functional class III or IV heart failure,[18] hypersensitivity, T1DM, DKA.
Adverse reactions	Upper respiratory tract infection, headache, sinusitis, pharyngitis, myalgia, edema, weight gain, dyspnea, macular edema.
Pregnancy	Category C. It use in lactation is unsafe.

Abbreviations: ALT, alanine aminotransferase; DKA, diabetic ketoacidosis; T1DM, type 1 diabetes mellitus.

Following are the synthetic GLP-1 receptor agonists available to treat diabetes. Short-acting GLP-1 receptor agonists (such as exenatide and lixisenatide) lower postprandial glucose levels and insulin concentrations by slowing gastric emptying. Long-acting GLP-1 receptor agonists (such as albiglutide, dulaglutide, exenatide long-acting release and liraglutide) predominantly lower blood glucose levels through stimulation of insulin secretion and reduction of glucagon levels.[21] Exenatide is a 39-amino acid peptide incretin mimetic that has glucoregulatory modes of actions similar to those of endogenous GLP-1.[22] Liraglutide increases intracellular cyclic adenosine monophosphate, which cause insulin release when blood sugar levels are elevated, it is a once-daily injectable GLP-1 receptor agonist and is not indicated as a first-line therapy. Dulaglutide, albiglutide is a once-weekly GLP-1 receptor agonist. Lixisenatide is dosed daily and is currently available as a combination medicine with insulin glargine (Soliqua; **Table 6**).

Dipeptidyl Peptidase 4 Inhibitors

DPP-4 inhibitors lower blood sugar levels by inhibiting DPP-4 and thereby stimulating levels of GLP-1 and other incretin hormone and prolong their action. They increase insulin release and decrease glucagon levels based on levels of glucose.[6] DPP-4 is as efficient as other known oral antidiabetic drugs, and is safer than sulfonylureas when comparing the incidence of hypoglycemic events; therefore, they are preferable to use older populations.[23] Sitagliptin can be used as a monotherapy or in combination with metformin or a thiazolidinedione. Linagliptin is a DPP-4 inhibitor that increases and prolongs incretin hormone activity. All DPP-4 are generally well-tolerated. They can be taken with or without food, but bioavailability is better if taken with food (**Table 7**).

Table 6
Glucagonlike peptide-1 agonists

Agent	Comment
Exenatide (Byetta) exenatide extended release (Bydureon)	
Dosage forms and strengths	As injectable solution, (Byetta) prefilled pen. 250 µg/mL, (1.2 mL vial). 250 µg/mL (2.4 mL vial). As injectable suspension (Bydureon). 2 mg/vial. 2 mg/syringe pen.
Initiation and maintenance	Immediate-release (Byetta): start 5 µg SC every 12 h within 60 min before meal, after 1 mo, may increase to 10 µg every 12 h. Extended release: Bydureon: 2 mg SC once weekly.
Dosing modifications	Moderate renal impairment: (CrCl 30–50 mL/min) caution when initiating or escalating dose. Avoid use if severe renal impairment (CrCl <30 mL/min) or ESRD.
Pharmacology	Half-life: 2.4 h (immediate release); 2 wk (extended release).
Liraglutide (Victoza)	
Dosage forms and strengths	Subcutaneous solution mulitidose pen18 mg/3 mL (Victoza) delivers doses of 0.6, 1.2, or 1.8 mg, 18 mg/3 mL.
Initiation and maintenance	Initiate Victoza: 0.6 mg SC daily for 1 wk, then increase to 1.2mg/d; if acceptable glycemic control not achieved then increase to 1.8 mg/d.
Dosing modifications	No adjustment necessary with renal and hepatic impairment.

(continued on next page)

Table 6
(continued)

Agent	Comment
Albiglutide (Tanzeum)	
Dosage Forms and Strengths	Lyophilized powder for reconstitution. 30 mg/pen. 50 mg/pen. Available as a single-use injectable pen.
Initiation and maintenance	30 mg SC once weekly; may increase to 50 mg once weekly if glycemic response is inadequate.
Dosing modifications	No dosage adjustment required for renal and hepatic impairment.
Dulaglutide (Trulicity)	
Dosage forms and strengths	SC solution. Available in single dose prefilled syringe or pen. 0.75 mg/0.5 mL. 1.5 mg/0.5 mL.
Initiation and maintenance	Initial: 0.75 mg SC once weekly, may increase dose to 1.5 mg once week.
Dosing modifications	No dosage adjustment required for renal or hepatic impairment.
Lixisenatide (Adlyxin)	
Dosage forms and strengths	SC solution in prefilled pen. Start dose (green pen), 50 μg/mL in 3 mL prefilled pen, which has 14 doses of 10 μg/dose. Maintenance dose (burgundy pen) 100 μg/mL in 3 mL prefilled pen.
Initiation and maintenance	Starting dose: 10 μg subcutaneous daily for 14 d. Maintenance: increase dose to 20 μg SC daily starting on day 15.
Dosing modifications	Renal impairment: Severe (CrCl 15–29 mL/min): Data are limited. closely monitor for GI adverse effects and for changes in renal function. Renal failure (CrCl <15 mL/min): not recommended.
Common issues in GLP-1	
Precautions	Pancreatitis: patients should be monitored for unexplained, persistent, severe abdominal pain and vomiting and the medication discontinued if acute pancreatitis develops.
Contraindications	In long acting GLP-1 agonists (all except Byetta and lixisenatide) it is contraindicated if the patient has a history or family history of medullary thyroid cancer and multiple endocrine neoplasia syndrome type 2. It causes thyroid C-cell tumors at clinically relevant exposures in rats and mice.
Adverse reactions	Nausea, vomiting and diarrhea, injection site reactions, antibody formation and increased heart rate.
Pregnancy	Category C: excretion in milk unknown; so use with caution. Limited data available for the use of Dulaglutide and lixisenatide in pregnancy and lactation.

Abbreviations: CrCl, creatinine clearance; GI, gastrointestinal; SC, subcutaneously.

Amylinomimetic

These agents mimic endogenous amylin. Amylin affects blood sugar control through slowed gastric emptying, reduction of food intake, and regulation of postprandial

Table 7
Dipeptidyl peptidase 4 inhibitors

Agent	Comment
Sitagliptin (Januvia)	
Dosage forms and strengths	Available in tablet 25, 50, and 100 mg.
Initiation and maintenance	100 mg orally daily.
Dosing modifications	Renal impairment: CrCl 30–50 mL/min: 50 mg/d. CrCl <30 mL/min, ESRD regardless of hemodialysis: 25 mg/d.
Saxagliptin (Onglyza)	
Dosage forms and strengths	Available as tablet 2.5 and 5 mg.
Initiation and maintenance	2.5–5 mg orally daily.
Dosing modifications	Renal impairment: CrCl <50 mL/min: not to exceed 2.5 mg/d. ESRD requiring hemodialysis: not to exceed 2.5 mg/d administered after dialysis.
Linagliptin (Tradjenta)	
Dosage forms and strengths	Available as 5-mg tablet.
Initiation and maintenance	5 mg orally daily.
Dosing modifications	Hepatic or renal impairment: no dosage adjustment required.
Alogliptin (Nesina)	
Dosage forms and strengths	Available as tablet 6.25, 12.5, and 25 mg.
Initiation and maintenance	25 mg orally daily.

Dosing modifications	Renal impairment.
	Moderate impairment: decrease dose to 12.5 mg/d.
	Severe impairment or ESRD requiring hemodialysis:
	  6.25 mg/d, may administer without regard to the timing of
	  dialysis.

Common issues in dipeptidyl peptidase 4 inhibitors	
Precautions	

Contraindications	Hypersensitivity to drug, diabetes mellitus type 1, diabetic
	  ketoacidosis, creatinine clearance <50, and history of
	  pancreatitis.

Adverse reactions	Angioedema, urticaria, and other immune-mediated
	  dermatologic effects can occur; acute pancreatitis and
	  heart failure have been reported.

Pregnancy	Category: B; not known whether excreted in breast milk: use with caution.

Abbreviations: CrCl, creatinine clearance; ESRD, end-stage renal disease.

glucagon. Amylin is deficient in type 1 diabetes and relatively deficient in insulin-requiring T2DM.[24,25]

Pramlintide (Symlin, SymlinPen 120, SymlinPen 60)
This agent is a synthetic analogue of human amylin. Pramlintide is used for the treatment of type 1 diabetes or T2DM in combination with insulin. It is administered before mealtime in patients who have not achieved acceptable glucose control despite optimal insulin therapy. It helps to lower blood glucose levels after meals, lessens

fluctuation of blood glucose levels during the day, and helps to improve long-term control of glucose levels compared with insulin alone[24] (**Table 8**).

Selective Sodium-Glucose Transporter-2 Inhibitors

Sodium-glucose cotransporter 2 inhibitors (SGLT2) lower blood glucose by increasing the urinary glucose excretion by lowering the renal glucose threshold. This class of drugs lowers blood glucose independent of insulin levels and sensitivity. They rarely cause hypoglycemia unless administered with other therapies that cause hypoglycemia. SGLT2 inhibitors reduce weight and blood pressure.[26] The available SGLT2 inhibitors are canagliflozin, dapagliflozin, and empagliflozin. Empagliflozin is indicated to reduce the risk of cardiovascular death in adults with T2DM. Euglycemic diabetic ketoacidosis has been reported in patients with T2DM and type 1 diabetes mellitus taking an SGLT2. In these individuals, the absence of hyperglycemia delays diagnosis of the problem. Serum ketones should be checked in any patient with nausea, vomiting, or malaise while taking SGLT2 inhibitors. There has been an increase in leg and foot amputations in patients taking canagliflozin reported. There is an increased risk for hypoglycemia when used with insulin and insulin secretagogues. Dose-related increases in low-density lipoprotein cholesterol have been reported. SGLT2 increase urinary glucose excretion and can have positive urine glucose tests so use alternative methods to monitor glycemic control[26] (**Table 9**).

Table 8 Amylinomimetics	
Dosage forms and strengths	Available as injectable solution: 0.6 mg/mL pen injector: 15, 30, 45, 60, and 120 μg/dose.
Initiation and maintenance	Type 1 diabetes: initial: 15 μg SC immediately before major meals. Increase by 15 μg every 3 d if not significant nausea. Reduce postprandial short-acting insulin dose by 50%. Maintenance: 30–60 μg SC. Type 2 diabetes: Initial: 60 μg SC immediately before major meals. After 3–7 d increase to 120 μg before meals if not significant nausea. Reduce postprandial short-acting insulin dose by 50%. Maintenance: 60–120 μg SC.
Dosing modifications	Renal impairment: no adjustments necessary.
Pharmacology	Half-life: 48 min.
Common issues in amylinomimetics	
Precautions	Do not mix with insulin - administer the 2 separately. It can delay the absorption of concomitantly administered oral medications. Administer concomitant oral medication at least 1 h prior or 2 h after pramlintide.
Contraindications	Black Box Warnings: use of pramlintide with insulin is associated with an increased risk of insulin induced severe hypoglycemia (occurs within 3 h of pramlintide injection), particularly in patients with type 1 diabetes. Contraindicated in hypersensitivity, gastroparesis, and hypoglycemia unawareness, recurrent severe hypoglycemia requiring assistance during the past 6 mo, HbA1c >9%, poor compliance patients, and pediatric patients.
Adverse reactions	Gastrointestinal side effects like nausea and vomiting, anorexia, abdominal pain.
Pregnancy	Category: C. Unknown whether excreted in breast milk so use caution.

Abbreviation: SC, subcutaneously.

| Table 9 |
| Selective sodium-glucose transporter-2 inhibitors |

Agent	Comment
Canagliflozin (Invokana)	
Dosage forms and strengths	Available as tablet 100 and 300 mg.
Initiation and maintenance	Start 100 mg orally daily taken before the first meal of the day. May increase dose to 300 mg/d.
Dosing modifications	Renal impairment. GFR 45–59: do not give more than 100 mg/d. GFR <45: do not initiate canagliflozin. GFR <30: Contraindicated.
Pharmacology	Half-life: 10.6 h for 100-mg dose and 13.1 h for 300-mg dose.
Dapagliflozin (Farxiga)	
Dosage forms and strengths	Available as tablet 5 and 10 mg
Initiation and maintenance	Initial: 5 mg/d, take in morning with or without food. May increase to 10 mg/d.
Dosing modifications	Renal impairment: GFR <60: do not initiate. Not recommended with GFR that declines persistently between 30 and <60. GFR <30 mL/min: contraindicated.
Pharmacology	Elimination: half-life: 12.9 h.
Empagliflozin (Jardiance)	
Dosage forms and strengths	Available as tablet 10 and 25 mg.
Initiation and maintenance	Start 10 mg/d in the morning, taken with or without food may increase to 25 mg/d if needed and tolerated.
Dosing modifications	Renal impairment: GFR <45 mL/min: do not initiate. Discontinue if GFR persistently falls below 45 mL/min.
Pharmacology	Half-life: 12.4 h.
Common issues in selective sodium-glucose transporter-2 inhibitors	
Precautions	Correct volume depletion before starting, cautious use if congestive heart failure, renal insufficiency, concomitant drugs that can cause renal dysfunction.
Contraindications	Type 1 diabetes, in T2DM with an estimated glomerular filtration of <60 mL/min for dapagliflozin or <45 mL/min for canagliflozin, and empagliflozin.
Adverse reactions	Hypotension especially in those using diuretics, angiotensin-converting enzyme inhibitors, or angiotensin receptor blockers, acute kidney injury, bone fracture, hyperkalemia, hypersensitivity reactions, diabetic ketoacidosis, genital yeast infections, urinary tract infections.[18]
Pregnancy	Category: C. Unknown if distributed in human breast milk so it is advised to discontinue.

Abbreviations: GFR, glomerular filtration rate; T2DM, type 2 diabetes mellitus.

Table 10
Bile acid sequestrants

Colesevelam (WelChol)

Dosage forms and strengths	Available as 625 mg tablet, 1875 and 3750 powder for oral suspension.
Initiation and maintenance	Tablet: 1.875 g (3 tablets) every 12 h with meals or 3.75 g (6 tablets) orally once daily with a meal. Oral suspension: 1.875 g (½ packet) orally every 12 h or 3.75 g (1 packet) once daily, mixed with liquid.

Common issues in bile acid sequestrants

Precautions	Dysphagia, major GI surgery, triglycerides 300–500, gastro paresis, type 1 diabetes mellitus or diabetic ketoacidosis.
Contraindications	Bowel obstruction or risk of bowel obstruction, triglyceride level of >500 mg/dL, history of hypertriglyceridemia-induced pancreatitis and hypersensitivity.
Adverse reactions	Hypersensitivity, rash, oral blister, intestinal obstruction, fecal impaction, dysphagia, pancreatitis constipation nausea, vomiting, and hypertriglyceridemia.
Pregnancy	Category: B, this drug is not expected to be excreted in breast milk.

Abbreviation: GI, gastrointestinal.

Bile Acid Sequestrants

The mechanism of action of bile acid sequestrants in lowering blood glucose levels are not clearly understood. The possible mechanisms include reduced or slowed absorption of ingested carbohydrates, which prevents postprandial glucose excursions, and absorption of fat leading to weight reduction and improved glucose control.[27]

Colesevelam is approved by the US Food and Drug Administration as an adjunct to diet and exercise to improve glucose control in adults with T2DM. It is taken in combination with insulin or oral antidiabetic agents. It can reduce absorption of some drugs and nutrients so administer drugs 4 hours before colesevelam and it can decrease absorption of fat-soluble vitamins. It can cause a reduced International Normalized Ratio in patients receiving warfarin and can cause elevated thyroid-stimulating hormone levels in patients receiving thyroid hormone replacement therapy (**Table 10**).

Table 11
Antiparkinsonian agents, dopamine agonists

Bromocriptine (Cycloset)

Dosage forms and strengths	Available as 5-mg capsule and 0.8- and 2.5-mg tablet.
Initiation and maintenance	Start 0.8-mg tablet daily, increase weekly by 1 tablet until maximal tolerated daily dose of 1.6–4.8 mg is achieved

Common issues antiparkinsonian agents, dopamine agonists

Precautions	Renal and hepatic impairment, psychosis and use with concurrent antihypertensive.
Contraindications	Type 1 diabetes, syncopal migraine, diabetes ketoacidosis, hypersensitivity breast feeding.
Adverse reactions	Nausea, vomiting, fatigue, dizziness, headache, hypotension, syncope, somnolence, hypoglycemia.
Pregnancy	Category: B. Should not be used during lactation.

Antiparkinsonian Agents, Dopamine Agonists

Bromocriptine (Cycloset)

This quick-release formulation is the only bromocriptine product used to treat T2DM mellitus. It is indicated as an adjunct to diet and exercise to improve glucose control. Take within 2 hours after waking in the morning with food. Bromocriptine (Cycloset) is thought to act on circadian neuronal activities within the hypothalamus and decrease fasting and postprandial hyperglycemia without increasing insulin levels[28] (**Table 11**).

SUMMARY

Pharmacotherapy to treat diabetes has changed greatly owing to various drugs and drug classes available. There are 11 classes of noninsulin diabetes medications available in the United States to treat T2DM. Single drug and combination therapies are effective in improving glycemic control in patients with diabetes. Important properties of the antidiabetic agents play a role in the choice of that particular medication for individual patients. Selection of antidiabetic medications should be done carefully, based on its efficacy, impact on weight, hypoglycemia risk, potential side effects, cost, and patient preferences.

REFERENCES

1. Control CfD, Prevention. National diabetes statistics report: estimates of diabetes and its burden in the United States, 2014. Atlanta (GA): US Department of Health and Human Services; 2014.
2. Apovian CM, Bergenstal RM, Cuddihy RM, et al. Effects of exenatide combined with lifestyle modification in patients with type 2 diabetes. Am J Med 2010;123(5): 468.e9-17.
3. Vancampfort D, Mitchell AJ, Hert M, et al. Type 2 diabetes in patients with major depressive disorder: a meta-analysis of prevalence estimates and predictors. Depress Anxiety 2015;32(10):763–73.
4. Feinkohl I, Price JF, Strachan MW, et al. The impact of diabetes on cognitive decline: potential vascular, metabolic, and psychosocial risk factors. Alzheimers Res Ther 2015;7(1):46.
5. Portillo-Sanchez P, Bril F, Maximos M, et al. High prevalence of nonalcoholic fatty liver disease in patients with type 2 diabetes mellitus and normal plasma aminotransferase levels. J Clin Endocrinol Metab 2015;100(6):2231–8.
6. Garber A, Abrahamson M, Barzilay J, et al. AACE/ACE consensus statement consensus statement by the American Association of Clinical Endocrinologists and American College of Endocrinology on the comprehensive type 2 diabetes management algorithm–2016 executive summary. 84. Endocr Pract 2016;22(1): 84–113.
7. Marathe PH, Gao HX, Close KL. American Diabetes Association standards of medical care in diabetes 2017. J Diabetes 2017;9(4):320–4.
8. Inzucchi SE, Bergenstal RM, Buse JB, et al. Management of hyperglycemia in type 2 diabetes: a patient-centered approach. Diabetes Care 2012;35(6): 1364–79.
9. Bailey CJ, Turner RC. Metformin. N Engl J Med 1996;334(9):574–9.
10. Kopecky C. Use of noninsulin antidiabetic medications in hospitalized patients. Crit Care Nurs Clin North Am 2013;25(1):39–53.
11. Kabadi MU, Kabadi UM. Efficacy of sulfonylureas with insulin in type 2 diabetes mellitus. Ann Pharmacother 2003;37(11):1572–6.

12. Wright A, Burden AF, Paisey RB, et al. Sulfonylurea inadequacy. Diabetes care 2002;25(2):330–6.
13. Guardado-Mendoza R, Prioletta A, Jiménez-Ceja LM, et al. The role of nateglinide and repaglinide, derivatives of meglitinide, in the treatment of type 2 diabetes mellitus. Arch Med Sci 2013;9(5):936.
14. Tornio A, Niemi M, Neuvonen M, et al. The effect of gemfibrozil on repaglinide pharmacokinetics persists for at least 12 h after the dose: evidence for mechanism-based inhibition of CYP2C8 in vivo. Clin Pharmacol Ther 2008; 84(3):403–11.
15. McCulloch D. Alpha-glucosidase inhibitors and lipase inhibitors for treatment of diabetes mellitus. Wolters Kluwer Health Clinical Solutions; 2007. Available at: https://www.uptodate.com/contents/alpha-glucosidase-inhibitors-and-lipase-inhibitors-for-treatment-of-diabetes-mellitus. Accessed July 31, 2017.
16. Lebovitz HE. Alpha-glucosidase inhibitors. Endocrinol Metab Clin North Am 1997;26(3):539–51.
17. Jonas D, Van Scoyoc E, Gerrald K, et al. Drug class review: newer diabetes medications, TZDs, and combinations. Available at: http://derp.ohsu.edu/about/final-document-display.cfm. Accessed July 31, 2017.
18. Inzucchi SE, Bergenstal RM, Buse JB, et al. Management of hyperglycemia in type 2 diabetes, 2015: a patient-centered approach: update to a position statement of the American Diabetes Association and the European Association for the study of diabetes. Diabetes Care 2015;38(1):140–9.
19. Ahrén B. Incretin dysfunction in type 2 diabetes: clinical impact and future perspectives. Diabetes Metab 2013;39(3):195–201.
20. Buse JB, Rosenstock J, Sesti G, et al. Liraglutide once a day versus exenatide twice a day for type 2 diabetes: a 26-week randomised, parallel-group, multinational, open-label trial (LEAD-6). Lancet 2009;374(9683):39–47.
21. Meier JJ. GLP-1 receptor agonists for individualized treatment of type 2 diabetes mellitus. Nat Rev Endocrinol 2012;8(12):728–42.
22. Gao Y, Yoon KH, Chuang LM, et al. Efficacy and safety of exenatide in patients of Asian descent with type 2 diabetes inadequately controlled with metformin or metformin and a sulphonylurea. Diabetes Res Clin Pract 2009;83(1):69–76.
23. Dicker D. DPP-4 inhibitors: impact on glycemic control and cardiovascular risk factors. Diabetes Care 2011;34(Suppl 2):S276–8.
24. Schmitz O, Brock B, Rungby J. Amylin agonists: a novel approach in the treatment of diabetes. Diabetes 2004;53(Suppl 3):S233–8.
25. Buse JB, Weyer C, Maggs DG. Amylin replacement with pramlintide in type 1 and type 2 diabetes: a physiological approach to overcome barriers with insulin therapy. Clin Diabetes 2002;20(3):137–44.
26. Miller E, Shubrook JH. Sodium glucose co-transporter 2 inhibitors in the treatment of type 2 diabetes mellitus. Osteopathic Fam Physician 2015;7(5):10–30.
27. Staels B, Kuipers F. Bile acid sequestrants and the treatment of type 2 diabetes mellitus. Drugs 2007;67(10):1383–92.
28. DeFronzo RA. Bromocriptine: a sympatholytic, D2-dopamine agonist for the treatment of type 2 diabetes. Diabetes Care 2011;34(4):789–94.

Insulin Therapy

The Old, the New and the Novel—An Overview

Veronica J. Brady, PhD, MSN, FNP-BC, BC-ADM, CDE[1]

KEYWORDS

- Diabetes • Type 2 diabetes • Insulin therapy • Novel therapy • Special populations

KEY POINTS

- The primary role of insulin therapy is to address the defect of β-cell failure.
- The goal of insulin therapy is to mimic normal insulin physiology.
- Although new and novel insulin formulations are available, there is still a role for neutral protamine Hagedorn and Regular insulin in diabetes management.
- Use of newer basal insulin formulations results in prolonged insulin action times and less hypoglycemia.
- Special considerations need be made when evaluating insulin therapy for older adults, pregnant women, persons with gastroparesis or those who are post gastric bypass.

INTRODUCTION

Diabetes is a group of diseases characterized by insufficient insulin production or inappropriate use. According to Dr Defronzo,[1] the pathophysiology of the disease is composed of etiologic mechanisms, which he refers to as the ominous octet. The octect consists of β-cell failure, decreased peripheral glucose use (muscle), increased hepatic glucose production (liver), adipocyte insulin resistance, increased glucagon secretion (α-cell), reduced incretin secretion and sensitivity (gastrointestinal), central nervous system insulin resistance from neurotransmitter dysfunction (brain), and enhanced glucose reabsorption (kidney).[1]

From the early days of the triumvirate to the current time of the ominous octet, β-cell decline leading to decreased insulin production has played a dominant role in diabetes. The total lack of insulin or impairment in production eventually leads to the need for exogenous insulin.

The author has no conflicts of interest to disclose.
University of Nevada, Reno School of Medicine, Reno, NV 89557, USA
[1] 1664 North Virginia, Suite 153, CMM 230, Reno, NV 89557.
E-mail address: vbrady@med.unr.edu

Type 2 diabetes mellitus (T2DM) affects approximately 29 million people (9.3% of the population) in the United States.[2] The cost of care is increasing consistently. Factors associated with cost of care include treatment of diabetes complications owing to poor glycemic control. Knowing that T2DM is a progressive disease leading to the requirement for insulin therapy over time would suggest that increasing numbers of patients will be on insulin therapy. However, despite the increase in prevalence of diabetes from 1988 to 2004 by 382%, synthesis of National Health and Nutrition Examination Survey data by Selvin and colleagues[3] revealed that the proportion of patients on insulin therapy has remained essentially unchanged from 1988 to 2004 (30.3%) to 2005 to 2012 (29.1%).

Over the last century since its discovery, insulin has been instrumental in prolonging the life of persons with diabetes as well as improving the quality of life. From the initial isolation of insulin in 1921 to present-day innovations (**Table 1**), the elusive goal has been to more closely approximate normal insulin physiology. Insulin was referred to by Cefalu and colleagues[4] as the "black dress"—that item that is essential, goes with everything and can be accessorized for any occasion. According to Owens and colleagues,[5] the lives of an estimated 5.1 million persons with type 1 diabetes worldwide were prolonged by approximately 1.5 years in 2000 alone. It was reported that, in 2001, more than 300 insulin analogues had been produced (although all have not reached the market), with more to come.[6] With all of the insulins currently available in the United States[7] (**Table 2**), how does one decide what insulin to use, when to use it, and in what patient, to get the best possible results?

NORMAL INSULIN PHYSIOLOGY

Plasma glucose levels in healthy individuals fluctuate within a very narrow range (63–126 mg/dL) despite nutritional intake, exercise, and other iatrogenic, physiologic, and

| Table 1 |
| The history of insulin |

Year	Type of Insulin	Manufacturer
1922	Pancreatic extraction for human use	Eli Lilly
1930	Neutral protamine Hagedorn (NPH)	Novo-Nordisk
1978–1982	Humulin R (rapid) and NPH	Genentech and Lilly
1996	Lispro	Lilly
2000	Aspart	Novo Nordisk
2000	Glargine	Sanofi
2004	Glulisine	Sanofi
2005	Detemir	Novo-Nordisk
2006	Exubera[a]	Sanofi and Pfizer
2014	Afrezza	Sanofi
2015	u-300 glargine	Sanofi
2015	u-200 Lispro	Lilly
2016	Degludec	Novo Nordisk
2016	Basaglar	Lilly
1952/1994	u-500 regular	Lilly

[a] No longer available.

Data from Quianzon CC, Cheikh I. History of insulin. J Community Hosp Intern Med Perspect 2012;2(2). doi: 10.3402/jchimp.v2i2.18701.

Table 2
Insulins available in the United States

Generic	Brand	Manufacturer	Form	Onset	Peak	Duration	Available Delivery	Storage
The old								
NPH	Humulin N Novolin N ReliOn N	Eli Lilly NovoNordisk	Human	1–3 h	4–8 h	12–16 h	10 mL vial, 3 mL KwikPen (5/box) 10 mL vial, 3 mL penfill (5/box) 10 mL vial	Refrigerate
Regular	Humulin R Novolin R ReliOn R	Eli Lilly NovoNordisk	Human	30–60 min	2–4 h	5–8 h	10 mL vial, 3 mL cartridge	Refrigerate
The new								
Lispro	Humalog	Eli Lilly	Human	10–20 min	30–90 min	3–5 h	3 mL vial, 10 mL vial, KwikPen 3 mL (5/box), 3 mL cartridge (5/box),	Refrigerate unused In use 28 d
Aspart	Novolog	NovoNordisk	Analogue	10–20 min	30–90 min	3–5 h	10 mL vial, FlexPen 3 mL (5/box), 3 mL cartridge (5/box),	Refrigerate unused In use 28 d
Glulisine	Apidra	Sanofi	Analogue	10–20 min	30–90 min	3–5 h	10 mL vial, Solostar Pen (5/box), OptiClik 3 mL (5/box)	Refrigerate unused In use 28 d
Glargine	Lantus	Sanofi	Analogue	60–90 min	No peak (8–12 h not pronounced)	20–26 h	10 mL vial, 3 mL Solostar Pen (5/box), OptiClik mL (5/box)	Refrigerate unused In use 28 d

(continued on next page)

Table 2 (continued)

Generic	Brand	Manufacturer	Form	Onset	Peak	Duration	Available Delivery	Storage
Detemir	Detemir	NovoNordisk	Analogue	60–90 min	No peak (4–7 h not pronounced)	20–26 h (17.5 h reported)	10 mL vial, 3 mL Flextouch Pen	In use no refrigeration good 42 d
The novel								
Inhaled insulin	Afrezza	Sanofi	Human	10–20 min	12–15 min	3 h	4 U –blue 8 U-green 12 U-yellow (cartridges) 2 inhalers	In haler good for 15 d 1 month-fridge 10 d sealed and 3 d unopened
Regular U500	Humulin R u-500	Eli Lilly	Human	30 min	8 h	Up to 24 h	10 mL vial (10,000 U) 3 mL pen fill (1500 U)	In use do not refrigerate Good for 28 d
Lispro	Humalog U-200	Eli Lilly	Analogue	15 min	30–90 min	3–5 h	KwikPen, 3 mL (600 U), (2/box)	In use 28 day—do not refrigerate
Glargine U-300	Lantus U-300 Toujeo	Sanofi	Analogue	6 h	No peak	36 h	Pen: 1.5 mL (450 U) (3/box)	Pen in use good for 42 d
Degludec	Tresiba	NovoNordisk	Analogue	30–90 min	No peak	42 h	Prefilled pen u-100 (300 U) Prefilled pen u-200 (600 U)	In use do not refrigerate up to 48 d

Adapted from Diabetes forecast. 2015. Insulins Available in the United States. diabetes.org.

psychological determinants. Plasma glucose levels usually peak 30 to 60 minutes after meals before returning to baseline in 2 to 3 hours. Basal insulin is the continuous insulin production to compensate for liver glucose (during fasting). Whereas prandial insulin is made up of first phase insulin, which constitutes the rapid increase in serum insulin levels to inhibit glucagon release and therefore inhibit glycogenolysis, and second phase insulin to maintain normoglycemia postprandially[5,8] (**Fig. 1**). The primary goal of treatment of diabetes is the restoration of glucose to near normal states (normoglycemia). It is found that this can be done most successfully by mimicking normal insulin physiology. Thus began, and continues to be, the quest to find and produce the perfect basal and bolus insulin preparations to replace normal physiologic production.

IN THE BEGINNING...THE OLD
Basal

In 1922, insulin was initially isolated from the pancreas of pigs and rabbits and administered with syringes that had to be boiled and needles that had to be sharpened.[9] During these early days, supply fell short of demand and there was often a 25% variation in potency within the same lot. With the need to inject multiple times a day the impetus was to find a way to prolong the duration of action. In 1936, neutral protamine Hagedorn (NPH) was "born."[10] In the 96 years since the successful extraction of insulin by Banting, Best, Collip, and Macleod, insulin has remained the mainstay of treatment for patients with type 1 diabetes mellitus and a fundamental part of treatment in T2DM.[10] NPH is considered to be the first basal insulin; however, it is actually intermediate acting insulin and is the only "basal" human insulin available.[11] NPH has an onset of action of 1 to 3 hours with a peak in approximately 8 hours and duration of action of 12 to 16 hours; however, the duration of action can vary significantly between patient and within the same patient, lasting 8 to 24 hours.[8]

Initiation
One of the most common ways of initiating NPH insulin is a regimen called BIDS (bedtime insulin daytime sulfonylureas; **Fig. 2**). This strategy involves continuing the patient on full-dose sulfonylureas and secretagogues during the day and adding a dose of NPH at night based on body weight (0.1–0.2 U/kg/d).[12,13] With the goal being to titrate the dose of NPH until the morning blood glucose is within target.

Caution
Some of the primary concerns with the use of NPH are that (1) patients must be instructed to mix the drug appropriately, and (2) they must be instructed on the timing of an injection. If not mixed appropriately, the pharmacokinetics of the drug will be distorted, leading to inconsistent active insulin profiles.[4] The other concern is for hypoglycemia. If the patient doses with dinner, they run the risk of early morning hypoglycemia; thus, the patient must be advised to eat a bedtime snack.

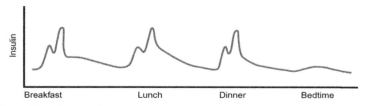

Fig. 1. Normal insulin secretion.

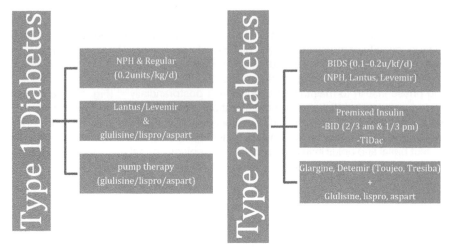

Fig. 2. Suggested insulin regimen. BID, 2 times a day; BIDS, bedtime insulin daytime sulfonylureas.

Benefits
The greatest benefit of NPH is that it is lower in cost and is available over the counter at some local pharmacies for $25 to $36 per vial.

Availability
Available formulations are Humulin N, Novolin N, and Relion N, which come in 10 mL vials.

Bolus

The oldest bolus insulin on the market is Regular. Regular insulin was developed from 1978 to 1982.[10] It was designed to be given 30 to 60 minutes before a meal in an effort to match the prandial spikes in blood glucose. The usual onset of action is between 2 and 4 hours with an expected peak in 5 to 8 hours.

Initiation
Regular insulin traditionally has been given (0.1 U/kg or 10% of basal dose) with largest meal of the day.[13]

Caution
The caution with regular insulin is that, owing to its longer action time, it should not be given after the meal.

Benefits
It too is inexpensive and available over the counter at the local pharmacy.

Availability
The available formulations include Humulin R, Novolin R, and Relion R, which come in 10 mL vials.

AS TIME GOES ON...THE NEW
Basal

Glargine
In 2000, glargine insulin came to market as a long-acting basal insulin. Glargine is produced using a nonpathogenic strain of *Escherichia coli*.[14] It is a human insulin

analogue that is soluble at an acidic pH of 4.0 and precipitates in subcutaneous tissue, leading to delayed absorption and extended duration of action. Glargine is reported to have duration of action of up to 24 hours with no reported accumulations after repeated injections (no stacking). It has an onset of action of 1 hour and a peakless profile. Thus, glargine does not cause the glycemic variability that was seen with NPH.[11]

Initiation It is given as a single daily injection, with usual starting doses of 10 U/d.

Benefits The incidence of hypoglycemia with glargine was found to be far less than that of NPH. Unlike NPH, it requires no rolling or shaking before administration.

Availability Glargine is available in 10 mL vials or 3 mL prefilled pens.

Detemir
Detemir insulin followed 5 years later. In 2005, NovoNordisk received approval for the second basal insulin. Detemir reversibly binds with albumin, thus prolonging the duration of action.[11]

Initiation As with other basal insulins, the usual starting dose is either 10 U or 0.1 to 0.2 U/kg/d.[13]

Benefits It has been found to be weight neutral.

Cautions In the experience of this author, in small doses (<20 U) Detemir has been found to have duration of action of 16 to 18 hours, thus requiring administration twice a day. This author has also noted that in some patients, there is a peak effect at about 2 to 3 hours, which may cause overnight hypoglycemia if bedtime blood glucose is less than 120 mg/dL.

Availability Detemir is available in 10 mL vials or 3 mL flextouch pens.

Bolus

In 1996 to 2005, a new era was ushered in for insulin therapy. During this time, insulin analogues came into play. Thus began the days of rapid-acting insulin and long-acting basal insulins.

Lispro
The first rapid-acting analogue on the scene was insulin Lispro produced by Eli Lilly in 1996. This insulin was new and exciting in that its onset is more rapid compared with human insulins, thus allowing for injection closer to the meal. When injected just before meals, they suppress postprandial glucose excursions.[5] The onset of action is 15 to 30 minutes with a peak of 30 to 60 minutes and action time of 3 to 4 hours.[11]

Aspart
Aspart, manufactured by Novo Nordisk, came to market in 2000. Aspart is structurally identical to human insulin[11] and has an onset, peak, and duration of action similar to that of Lispro.

Glulisine
Glulisine was the last rapid-acting insulin to market in 2004. It is produced using nonpathogenic *E coli* by recombinant DNA technology. Glulisine has onset, peak, and duration times similar to those of the other two rapid-acting insulins.

Benefits

Even when injected up to 15 minutes after the meal, these analogues are as effective as their human counterparts taken 30 minutes before meals. The analogues also allow for greater flexibility in timing of meals and cause less overnight hypoglycemia. With the unique property of being approved for administration after the meal, Glulisine is the prandial insulin of choice for patient experiencing nausea and vomiting, that is, those with gastroparesis or undergoing treatment for cancer (chemotherapy, radiation therapy, etc).

Availability

All of the rapid acting insulins are available in 10 mL vials or 3 mL prefilled syringes.

UP UNTIL NOW...THE NOVEL

U300 Glargine

In 2015, U-300 glargine became available (**Table 3**). This product is a formulation of glargine with 300 U/mL. This allows for the same amount of insulin to be delivered with one-third of the volume. U-300 glargine has a longer duration of action (36 hours), no peak, and was found to decrease risk of hypoglycemia. It also leads to less weight gain. This basal insulin is designed for use in patients with extreme insulin resistance (requiring >200 U/d). The pen device will accommodate up to 80 U as a single injection.[15] It is available in prefilled pen with 1.5 mL (450 U).

Degludec

Insulin degludec is one of the newest weapons in our arsenal for use in the fight against diabetes. It became available in 2016. Degludec is an ultra–long-acting insulin analogue that binds to albumin and has duration of action of 42 hours. It has no appreciable peak and produces a stable glucose-lowering affect. Degludec causes less nocturnal hypoglycemia than glargine.[16] This lengthy duration of action allows for flexibility in administration on the part of the patient. Degludec is available in both U-100 and U-200 concentrations. It comes in a prefilled pen: U-100 with 300 U and U-200 with 600 U. It also has the added benefit of providing up to 160 U as a single

Table 3
Novel insulin considerations

Insulin	Concentration	Benefits	Considerations
U-300 glargine (Toujeo)	U300	Smaller volume Less hypoglycemia Longer duration of action	No conversions needed
Degludec (Tresiba)	U100/U200	Longer duration of action—with flexibility in timing of doses Less hypoglycemia Smaller volume available	May need dose adjustment when switching from u100 basal
U-500 Humulin R	U500	Meets basal and prandial needs Dose 2 or 3 times a day	Use pen fill devices or u500 syringes, which require no dose conversion
U-200 Humalog	U200	Smaller volume	No conversions needed
Inhaled insulin (Afrezza)	U100	Inhaled—no injections	Check pulmonary function tests Set doses only (4,8,12 U)

dose. The use of this insulin is ideal for those patients on the go who often have reported missing a dose of insulin owing to their schedules or an inability to remember. Because there is no reported "stacking" effect, the timing of the insulin is not crucial. Also, those patients with substantial insulin needs, but not desiring to perform more than 1 basal injection, have the ability to administer a larger single injection with a small volume (using U-200) is beneficial.

U-500 Regular

U-500 Humulin regular insulin—what is old is new again

U-500 Regular insulin was first available in 1952. Most recently, we have seen resurgence in its use. It is primarily used for patients who are extremely insulin resistant (requiring > 200 U/d). There is a 5-fold greater concentration of insulin in U-500 Regular insulin compared with U-100 insulin, leading to a delayed peak and longer duration of action. It is reported to peak in 8 hours with a duration of action up to 24 hours. In the past, U-500 Regular insulin prescriptions needed to be written to include both the insulin dose and volume (100 U = 0.2 mL = 20 U on u100 syringe).[17] Today, U-500 Humulin R is available in a 3 mL prefilled pen (1500 U) or 20 mL vial to be used with a U-500 insulin syringe.

Inhaled Insulin

The most novel insulin formulation of all—inhaled insulin, was reintroduced in 2014. The last inhaled insulin on the market, Exubera, was introduced in 2006, but did not fare well. The latest entry into the arena is Afrezza. Afrezza is a finely powered inhaled insulin that has an onset of action in 10 to 20 minutes, peaks in 12 to 15 minutes, and has a duration of action of about 3 hours.[9] It is not recommended for use in patients who smoke or have recently stopped smoking, have kidney disease, or are pregnant. Before prescribing patients should have pulmonary function test (FEV_1). It is available in 4, 8, or 12 U cartridges—thus, if other doses are needed, combinations of cartridges will need to be used.

Others

The other 2 drugs in the novel category are basaglar and U-200 Humalog. Basaglar is biosimilar to glargine and has properties that are similar. U-200 Humalog has the properties of Humalog and is primarily useful in patients with extreme insulin resistance requiring greater doses of insulin owing to the fact that one-half of the volume is administered.

BACK TO THE FUTURE—WHAT'S NEXT
Soliqua

In the quest to improve glycemic control, the search for better, more effective treatment options is never ending. The most recent developments are the combinations of a basal insulin with a glucagon-like peptide-1. Early in 2017, Sanofi brought Soliqua 100/33 to market. Soliqua was approved by the US Food and Drug Administration in 2016 and is a combination of glargine 100 U and lixisenatide 33 μg/mL.

Population

It is designed for use in patients with T2DM requiring less than 60 U of basal insulin per day or lixisenatide, but not yet meeting their hemoglobin A1c goal.

Initiation

For patients meeting these criteria, Soliqua is initiated at 15 U (15 U glargine/5 µg lixisenatide) subcutaneously once a day 1 hour before the first meal of the day in patient on less than 30 U of basal insulin per day. For those on 30 to 60 U of basal insulin, the starting dose is 30 U (30 U glargine/10 µg lixisenatide). The maximum dose is 60 U (60 U glargine/20 µg lixisenatide).

Availability

The drug is available in 3 mL prefilled pens.

Xultophy

The other combination drug in this class is Xultophy 100/3.6 (insulin degludec and liraglutide).

Population

The indication for use is in patients with T2DM inadequately controlled on less than 50 U of basal insulin daily or liraglutide less than 1.8 mg/d.

Initiation

To start, degludec and liraglutide must be discontinued. The starting dose is 16 U (16 U degludec and liraglutide 0.58) subcutaneously daily, independent of food. The maximum dose is 50 U (50 U degludec/1.8 mg liraglutide).

Availability

The drug is available in 3 mL prefilled pen.

Benefits

One benefit is that the patient is only required to take one injection daily to get the benefit of both a basal insulin and glucagon-like peptide-1. Another benefit is that this combination may decrease the amount of weight gain that is often associated with insulin therapy.

Cautions

The primary concern with use of this drug is that it has dose limitations and titration is required to get to maximum dose of glucagon-like peptide-1.

SPECIAL POPULATIONS

As with all medications, there is always an exception to the rule and with insulin therapy things are no different. A couple of the special populations to take into consideration are insulin pumpers, pregnant women, older adults, post bariatric surgery patients, and those with gastroparesis.

- Pumpers: Often, those with an insulin pump need to be reminded to discontinue basal insulin once they begin on pump therapy. Also, several of the pump companies do not recommend the use of Glulisine in the pumps owing to believed instability after 2 days. U-200 Humalog and U-500 regular have been used in pumps on occasion, but this is not the standard of care.
- Pregnant women: not all insulins are recommended for use during pregnancy (**Table 4**). The benefits should outweigh the risks to the fetus when prescribing. NPH and regular or Detemir and Humalog are the insulins most often used in pregnancy.
- Older adults: When prescribing for older adults, one must take into consideration dietary intake, cost, complexity of regimen, and patient functional and cognitive

Table 4
Insulin safety in pregnancy

Drug	Safety Category
Lantus	C
Detemir	B
NPH	B
Regular	B
Lispro	B
Aspart	B
Glulisine	C
Tresiba	C
Toujeo	C
Afrezza	

B, animal studies have shown no adverse effects no adequate well controlled studies in pregnant women; C, animal studies have shown some adverse events, no adequate well controlled studies in pregnant women. Use only if benefits outweigh risks.

status, as well as other comorbid conditions. The goal of therapy should be tailored to life expectancy and perceived burden to the patient. When considering basal insulin therapy, it has been reported that glargine causes fewer hypoglycemic events than Detemir.

- Post bariatric surgery patients: After surgery, the expectation is that the patient will have fairly rapid weight loss, thus leading to decreased insulin resistance and decreased insulin needs. These patients will likely require rapid insulin adjustments and need to monitor carefully for hypoglycemia.
- Gastroparesis: Gastroparesis is a challenging situation, depending on where the patient is along the spectrum. It may often be advisable to have the patient take the insulin after the meal; therefore, Glulisine may be the recommended prandial insulin. Regular insulin may also be considered owing to the delayed gastric emptying; it may be better suited to combating postprandial blood glucose fluctuations.

OTHER CONSIDERATIONS

In prescribing insulin therapy, there are many things to consider.

- Cost of the insulin: Can the patient afford the newer insulins? Would they be better served with an older insulin regimen that they can get for a fraction of the cost? Do they have insurance coverage and, if so, does their insurance plan dictate which insulin they can get at tier 1 cost verses tier 3.
- Manual dexterity and visual acuity: Will the patient be able to withdraw the insulin from a vial using a syringe or would they be better served with a pen device? Are they able to read the numbers on the pen device and depress the plunger effectively?
- Length of pen needle: Is the patient thin? Will use of a 12 mm needle result in the insulin being administered intramuscularly? Are they obese, requiring larger doses of insulin and use of a 4 mm needle will result in leakage after the injection? Frid and colleagues[18] offer detailed recommendations on insulin delivery.

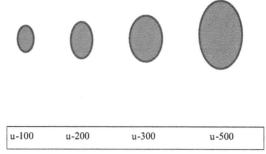

| u-100 | u-200 | u-300 | u-500 |

Fig. 3. Volume comparison based on insulin concentration.

- Volume of syringe: How much insulin are they injecting? How difficult is it to determine the amount of insulin using a 1 mL syringe when the required insulin dose is 12 U?
- Large doses of insulin: Those using greater than 200 U of insulin a day would likely be best served by the use of U-200, U-300, or U-500 insulins (**Fig. 3**). The decrease in volume will often lead to increased or improved insulin absorption.

SUMMARY

Insulin therapy will always be a necessity in the lives of people with type 1 diabetes mellitus as a first-line therapy and it is often last line for those with T2DM and progressive β-cell failure. One of the things to consider when your patient has not reached their hemoglobin A1c goal is that only 70% of the patients who are prescribed insulin therapy are actually taking it within the appropriate timeframe.[19] Thus, the first thing to do would be to evaluate adherence before intensifying therapy. When the decision is made to initiate or intensify therapy, the challenge will be to decide which insulin to use

Table 5 Premixed insulins					
Generic	Brand Name	Onset (min)	Peak	Duration (h)	Available Delivery
70%NPH/30% Regular	Humulin 70/30	30–60	Varies	10–16	10 mL vial, 3 mL prefilled pen (5/box)
70%NPH/30% Regular	Novolin 70/30	30–60	Varies	10–16	10 mL vial, 3 mL prefilled cartridge (5/box)
70%NPH/30% Regular	ReliOn 70/30	30–60	Varies	10–16	10 mL vial
50%NPH/50% Regular	Humulin 50/50	30–60	Varies	10–16	10 mL vial
75%lispro protamine/ (NPL)/25% insulin Lispro	Humalog 75/25	10–15	Varies	10–16	10 mL vial, 3 mL KwikPen (5/box)
50%lispro protamine/50 insulin Lispro	Humalog 50/50	10–15	Varies	10–16	10 mL vial, 3 mL KwikPen (5/box)
70% Aspart protamine/ 30% Aspart	Novolog Mix 70/30	5–15	Varies	10–16	10 mL vial, 3 mL FlexPen (5/box)

under which circumstances. The American Diabetes Association has provided detailed algorithms on the initiation of insulin.[13] Once daily basal insulin is the easiest to start, with progression to multiple dose insulin as insulin needs increase. If patients have consistent dietary intake and desire a simplified regimen premixed insulin (**Table 5**) may be feasible. Patients with extreme insulin resistance will likely benefit from concentrated insulin preparations, that is, U-200 Humalog, U-300 glargine, or U-500 Humulin R. Keep in mind that the overall goal of therapy is to improve glycemic control, thereby decreasing diabetes complications.

REFERENCES

1. Defronzo R. Overview of newer agents: where treatment is going. Am J Med 2010;123:S38–48.
2. American Diabetes Association. Fast facts-data and statistics about diabetes. 2016. Available at: professional.diabetes.org/facts. Accessed May 7, 2017.
3. Selvin E, Parrinello CM, Daya N, et al. Trends in insulin use and diabetes control in the U.S.: 1988-1994 and 1999-2012. Diabetes Care 2016;36:e33–5.
4. Cefalu WT, Rosenstock J, LeRoith D, et al. Insulin's role in diabetes management: after 90 years still considered the essential "black dress". Diabetes Care 2015;38: 2200–3.
5. Owens DR, Zinman B, Bolli GB. Insulins today and beyond. Lancet 2001;358: 739–46.
6. Pillai O, Panchagnula R. Insulin therapies—past, present and future. Drug Discov Today 2001;6(20):1056–61.
7. Diabetes forecast. Insulins available in the United States. 2015. Available at: diabetes.org.
8. Pettus J, Cavaiola TS, Tamborlane WV, et al. The past, present and future of basal insulins. Diabetes Metab Res Rev 2016;32:478–96.
9. Curry A. Insulin innovations: new forms of insulin at your pharmacy and on the horizon. 2015. Available at: http://www.diabetesforecast.org/2015/jul-aug/insu-lin-innovations.html. Accessed May 15, 2016.
10. Quianzon CC, Cheikh I. History of insulin. J Community Hosp Intern Med Per-spect 2012;2(2). http://dx.doi.org/10.3402/jchimp.v2i2.18701.
11. Kiara S. Advances in insulin therapy. 2013. Available at: http://jpma.org/Abou-tUs.php. Accessed May 13, 2017.
12. Edelman SV. A practical approach to combination therapy: daytime oral agent(s) and bedtime NPH insulin. Clin Diabetes 1999;7(3):100. Available at: http://journal.diabetes.org/clinicaldiabetes/V17N31999/Pg100.htm.
13. American Diabetes Association Position Statement: standards of medical care in diabetes—2017. Diabetes Care 40(Suppl 1):S1–135.
14. McKeage K, Goa KL. Insulin glargine: a review of its therapeutic use as a long-acting agent for the management of type 1 and 2 diabetes mellitus. Drugs 2001; 61(11):1599.
15. White J. Advances in insulin therapy: a review of new insulin glargine 300 units/mL in the management of diabetes. Clin Diabetes 2016;34(2):86–91.
16. Zinman B. Newer insulin analog: advances in basal insulin replacement. Diabetes Obes Metab 2013;15(Suppl 1):6–10.
17. Dailey AM, Tannock LR. Extreme insulin resistance: indications and approaches to the use of u-500 insulin in type 2 diabetes mellitus. Curr Diab Rep 2010;11: 77–82.

18. Frid AH, Kreugel G, Grassi G, et al. New insulin delivery recommendations. Mayo Clin Proc 2016;91(9):1231–55.
19. Gale EA. Newer insulins in type 2 diabetes. BMJ 2012;345:44–8.

A Primer on Insulin Pump Therapy for Health Care Providers

Deborah L. McCrea, MSN, RN, FNP-BC, CNS, CEN, CFRN, EMT-P

KEYWORDS

- Insulin pump • Basal and bolus rate
- Advantages/disadvantages/candidates selection/contraindications
- Troubleshooting insulin pumps

KEY POINTS

- Health care providers need to understand the advantages, disadvantages, candidate selection criteria, and contraindications for an insulin pump.
- Optional features such as variable bolus, and temporary and alternate basal patterns can help to achieve improved glycemic control.
- Troubleshooting insulin pump–related problems is imperative to minimize hypoglycemia, hyperglycemia, and diabetic ketoacidosis.
- All insulin pump companies have 24-h customer service and web support for the patient and health care provider.

INTRODUCTION

Currently, 375, 000 to 400,000 of the 3 million people in the United States with type 1 diabetes (T1DM) use an insulin pump. It is estimated that there may be more than 1 million people wearing an insulin pump worldwide, which is up from 130,000 in 2002. Approximately 6% of adults and 19% of children with T1DM use an insulin pump.[1–4]

WHAT IS AN INSULIN PUMP?

An insulin pump is a small, battery-powered, programmable device that delivers rapid-acting insulin in very small doses into a subcutaneous space to mimic the natural insulin release by the pancreatic beta cells. By dosing rapid acting insulin in a

Disclosure Statement: The author has nothing to disclose.
Department of Acute and Continuing Care, University of Texas Health Science Center at Houston, School of Nursing, 6901 Bertner Avenue, Suite 695, Houston, TX 77030, USA
E-mail address: Deborah.L.McCrea@uth.tmc.edu

Nurs Clin N Am 52 (2017) 553–564
http://dx.doi.org/10.1016/j.cnur.2017.07.005
0029-6465/17/© 2017 Elsevier Inc. All rights reserved.

more controlled manner, the user often has improved blood glucose (BG), increased flexibility, and improved quality of life. The health care provider needs to understand the advantages, disadvantages and candidate selection criteria so they can guide those patients wishing to get an insulin pump. The health care provider must then understand how to calculate and adjust starting insulin pump doses and how to troubleshoot for common insulin pump problems such as hypoglycemic and hyperglycemia.

INTENSIVE DIABETES CONTROL RESEARCH

The DCCT (Diabetes Control and Complications Trial) was a landmark trial conduced from 1983 to 1993 which showed that intensive insulin therapy reduced long-term diabetes complications compared with nonintensive insulin therapy in patients with T1DM. The findings revealed that intensive glucose control reduced retinopathy by 76%, nephropathy by 50%, and neuropathy by 60%. When the DCCT ended, a follow-up trail, the EDIC trial (Epidemiology of Diabetes Intentions and Complications) looked at stroke, myocardial infarction and heart surgery. Again, intensive therapy reduced cardiovascular disease events by 42% and nonfatal myocardial infarction, stroke, or death from cardiovascular disease by 57%. Both studies showed the benefit of intensive diabetes management in patients with T1DM[5-6] (**Table 1**).

HISTORY OF INSULIN PUMPS

Dr Arnold Kadish developed the first insulin pump prototype in 1963. He attempted to mimic pancreatic beta cell insulin delivery; however, the pump was the size of a backpack and delivered insulin intravenously rather than subcutaneously. In 1973, Dean Kamen developed the AS2C insulin pump, also called the "blue brick" because it had the same dimensions as a brick. Mr Kamen's next pump, the "autosyringe," was smaller and more discrete and was used to deliver a variety of medications. The first pump developed exclusively for insulin was from Minimed, Inc., in 1983. Since that time, pumps have become much smaller and have more programmable features.[8-13]

Table 1
Synopsis of the Diabetes Control and Complications Trial (DCCT) and Epidemiology of Diabetes Intentions and Complications Trial (EDIC)

Complications	DCCT (%)[a]	EDIC (%)[b]
Retinopathy: 3 step change	63	72
Retinopathy: proliferative	47	76
Retinopathy: macular edema	26	77
Retinopathy: laser therapy	51	77
Nephropathy: microalbuminuria	39	53
Nephropathy: clinical albuminuria	54	82
Neuropathy	60	—

Reduction in risk for microvascular complication with intensive therapy, compared with conventional therapy as demonstrated during the DCCT and EDIC trials.
  [a] $P<.4$ for all reductions, except for macular edema during DCCT, which was not significant.
  [b] EDIC assessment of neuropathy was different from DCCT assessment, precluding comparison of DCCT and EDIC results.[7]

SAFETY OF INSULIN PUMPS

The US Food and Drug Administration reported insulin pumps are generally safe in managing diabetes and that most adverse events were owing to operator error. Safety issues reported with insulin pumps include:

- Failing to notice disconnected infusion sets,
- Damaged pump from temperature and water,
- Not reconnecting pump after removal,
- Using an infusion set for more than 3 days,
- Reusing the same infusion sites frequently,
- Not testing BG levels as recommended,
- Overriding or improperly programming bolus calculator software,
- Forgetting to bolus for food or hyperglycemia, and
- Not carbohydrate counting correctly.[14,15]

ADVANTAGES AND DISADVANTAGES, AND CANDIDATE SELECTION AND CONTRAINDICATIONS
Advantages

Pump therapy is considered the gold standard for precise insulin delivery.[16] A survey found that 96% of diabetes specialists including physicians, nurse practitioners, physician assistants, and certified diabetes educators who have T1DM practice intensive insulin management for their own diabetes and more than one-half choose to wear an insulin pump.[17] The advantages include the following:

- Reduces need for insulin injections by syringe or pen,
- Delivers precise amounts of rapid-acting insulin,
- Reduces variability in BG levels,
- Allows for more precise dosing during growth spurts,
- Reduces severe hypoglycemia, especially at night,
- Reduces risk of long-term diabetes complications,
- Makes delivery of bolus insulin easier,
- Minimizes insulin stacking,
- Convenient lifestyle with flexibility,
- Variable bolus options for gastroparesis or high-fat meals,
- Temporary basal rates for exercise or prolonged fasting,
- Able to eat fewer carbohydrates for exercise to avoid extra calories,
- Easy tracking of data software,
- Ease of travel, especially through time zones,
- Ease for those with variable work or school schedules,
- Able to bolus insulin discreetly,
- Allows for easier weight loss by matching insulin to food intake, and
- Improved quality of life.[2,16,18–20]

Disadvantages

Although there are many benefits to wearing the insulin pump, the disadvantages include the following.

- An initial steep learning curve.
- Cost.
- Because the insulin pump only uses rapid- or short-acting insulin, severe hyperglycemia and diabetic ketoacidosis can develop quickly if there is any disruption of insulin delivery or insulin absorption, such as:

- Pump malfunction,
- Dead battery,
- Loss of the infusion set,
- Poor absorption of insulin from the infusion site, or
- Loss of insulin potency.

Candidate Selection

For pump therapy to be a positive and beneficial experience, the medical provider needs to carefully consider which candidate would benefit from insulin pump therapy. The ideal candidate would possess one or more of the following characteristics.

- Requires insulin therapy.
- Desires to use the insulin pump.
- Following a multiple daily insulin injection regimen.
- Motivated and willing to participate in self-management.
- Willing to check their BG levels throughout the day.
- Able to evaluate food choices.
- Able to problem solve.
- Supportive family members.
- Labile BG despite best efforts.
- Elevated hemoglobin A1c.
- Hypoglycemia unawareness.
- Recurrent or unpredictable hypoglycemia,
- Nocturnal hypoglycemia,
- Preconception or pregnancy.
- Dawn phenomena.
- Postmeal hyperglycemia.
- Erratic lifestyles, such as college students, shift workers, and frequent travelers.
- Intensive exercise.
- Gastroparesis
- Extreme insulin sensitivity or resistance.
- Early neuropathy or nephropathy.
- Renal transplantation.
- Can afford it.
- Capable intellectually, physically, and technically.
- Demonstrates emotional stability.
- Able to follow standard hypoglycemia and hyperglycemia protocols.[2,16,20–23]

Contraindications

If a patient has a contraindication to starting pump therapy, they may become a candidate in the future. The contraindications include the following.

- Not willing to perform BG checks.
- Does not want to use the insulin pump.
- Does not keep diabetes appointments,
- The patient or significant other is unable or unwilling to learn how to
  - Use the insulin pump,
  - Count carbohydrates and quantify food,
  - Carry emergency backup supplies,
  - Treat hypoglycemia including the use of glucagon, and
  - Troubleshoot hyperglycemia and prevention of diabetic ketoacidosis.

- Has evidence of psychiatric illness that will impede pump use.
- Lack of insurance or ability to pay for pump and supplies.[2]

PUMP MECHANICS, MODES, AND EQUIPMENT

All insulin pumps, except one have a disposable syringe known as a reservoir or cartridge that the patient fills with insulin and is connected to an infusion set that has a small catheter, which is manually placed into the subcutaneous skin. The catheter can be made of Teflon, metal or other materials. One brand does not have infusion set. The Omnipod has a built-in reservoir and catheter with an automatic inserter, delivery mechanism, and power supply. It has a remote controller to program the pump settings. Insulin pump sites are changed every 2 to 3 days. Each pump has a variety of features and functions from which to choose. Options include colors, alarms, delivery rates, reservoir sizes, infusion sets, cannula materials, cannula sizes, adhesives, and other features. A full comparison chart of current pumps as of March 2017 can be found at the following link: http://main.diabetes.org/dforg/pdfs/2017/2017-cg-insulin-pumps.pdf. See **Table 2** for the contact information for the insulin pump companies in the United States.

INSULIN FOR THE PUMP

Insulin pumps use rapid acting insulin such as Lispro, Aspart, Glulisine, or Regular insulin. Regular insulin is rarely used today owing to a slower onset when compared with insulin analogues. Rapid-acting insulin begins to work in as little as 5 to 15 minutes; Regular insulin has an onset of 30 minutes. This delay in insulin action can cause the BG to increase after ingesting carbohydrates if the bolus is given at the same time carbohydrate is consumed. Therefore, it is recommended to bolus 15 minutes before eating to avoid a postprandial meal spike, if using a rapid acting insulin and 30 minutes before eating if using Regular insulin. If the patient has gastroparesis or consumes high-fat meals, the bolus may need to be customized.

BASAL RATE

The purpose of the basal rate is to match the glucose being released from the liver during the fasting state. Delivered around the clock, the basal rate is programmed

Table 2		
Contact information on insulin pump companies in the United States		
Company	**Contact Information**	**Pumps**
Animas Corp	https://www.animas.com 877–937–7867	One Touch Ping Vibe
Insulet Corp	https://www.myomnipod.com 800–591–3455	Omnipod
Medtronic Diabetes	https://www.medtronicdiabetes.com 800–646–4633	MiniMed Paradigm Revel MiniMed 530G MiniMed 630G MiniMed 670G
Sooil	http://www.sooil.com 866–747–6645	Dana Diabecare R Dana Diabecare IIS
Tandem Diabetes Care	https://www.tandemdiabetes.com 877–801–6901	T-flex T:slim G4 T:slim x2

to maintain BG in target range between meals and while sleeping. This continual release of insulin takes the place of intermediate and long-acting insulin. The total basal dose is approximately 50% of the total daily pump dose.[2,24] Basal rates can be delivered in increments as small as 0.025 units per hour and as large as 35 units per hour for those who require very small or large basal doses, and can change rates every 30 minutes to match their metabolic needs.[18]

Many patients with diabetes have dawn phenomenon. Dawn phenomenon is caused when growth hormones, cortisol, and catecholamines are released in greater amounts to prepare the body to wake up in the morning causing the BG to increase between 2 a.m. and 8 a.m. The basal rate can be programmed to increase automatically to match insulin needs during that time of day. If the basal rate is set correctly, the user should be able to delay or a skip meal, or sleep longer than normal without developing hypoglycemia or hyperglycemia.

TEMPORARY BASAL RATES AND ALTERNATE BASAL PATTERNS

A temporary basal rate can be programmed from 0% to 200% from 30 minutes to 24 hours and is used for temporary issues such as:

- Sick days,
- Exercise and increased activity,
- Inactivity,
- Stress,
- Hormones,
- Medications than can change BG, and
- Prolonged fasting.[25]

Alternate basal patterns are preset basal rates than can be used when more or less insulin is needed for semiregular purposes. They can be preset ahead of time and simply switched on when needed. Many pumps have 2 to 3 alternate basal patterns that can be preprogrammed ahead of time. Common reasons that insulin pump users program alternate basal patterns include:

- Menstrual cycle,
- Steroids,
- Varying weekly events such as inactivity during the week and active on weekends,
- Exercise,
- Erratic schedules,
- Travel or camp, and
- Fasting for religious purposes, medical tests, procedures, or surgery.

BOLUS RATE

The bolus rate is the insulin delivered to cover carbohydrate intake and to correct hyperglycemia. It normally represents the other 50% of the daily insulin needs. Most meal or snack boluses should be given 15 minutes before eating to better match the onset of the rapid acting insulin and the rise in the BG from the carbohydrate digestion to avoid a postmeal spike in BG.

The bolus can be delivered all at once, or all slowly over a period of time, or a combination of part rapid and part slow delivery. The slow bolus delivery can be programmed from 30 minutes to 8 hours. Common reasons for delivering a slow or combination bolus includes eating at events where the food may be delivered slowly in courses such as banquets, buffets, and parties. High-fat meals increase insulin resistance after eating, which may cause hyperglycemia hours later, so a combination bolus may be needed. The BG may initially decrease and then increase after ingesting a high-protein and low-carbohydrate meal, so an extended or combination bolus may be needed. Patients with gastroparesis have delayed gastric motility and often require an extended bolus. Parents of young children who have unpredictable eating patterns often use a combination bolus so the bolus can be canceled if the child does not finish the meal. Frequent BG testing or the use of a continous glucose sensor monitor can help to identify which variable bolus is needed (**Table 3**).[2,22] There are many web sources to learn how to use the variable bolus feature including:

- https://www.diabetesalaska.com/diabetes_ip_bolusing.html
- https://www.diabetesdaily.com/blog/ids-article-297761/
- http://www.diabetesclinic.ca/en/diab/5pumps/profguide_instherapy.pdf
- https://s3.amazonaws.com/medtronic-hcp/Pumping%20Protocol%20-%20a% 20Guide%20to%20Insulin%20Pump%20Therapy%20Initiation.pdf
- https://myglu.org/articles/5-diabetes-meal-time-tips-from-medtronic
- http://clinidiabet.com/en/infodiabetes/pumps/23.htm
- https://www.baker.edu.au/-/media/Documents/fact-sheets/BakerIDI-HPfactsheet-extended-wave-bolus.ashx?la=en
- http://waltzingthedragon.ca/Split__Combo_Dual__Bolus.html
- www.medtronicdiabetes.com/sites/default/files/library/support/Basics%20of% 20Insulin%20Pump%20Therapy.pdf

BOLUS CALCULATORS

Many pumps on the market have built-in bolus calculators to determine the bolus dose. The BG can be manually entered into the pump or a linked glucose meter can automatically send the BG to the pump. The carbohydrate gram amount is manually

Table 3
Initial insulin pump settings
Step 1: Determine the initial total insulin pump dose. Can average both methods or start at the higher dose for elevated hemoglobin A1c or pregnancy, or at the lower value for those with hypoglycemia issues.
Method 1: Prepump total daily dose × 0.75 / Method 2: Weight kg × 0.5 or Weight pounds × 0.23
Step 2: Calculate the initial single basal rate based on step 1.   • Pump total daily dose × 0.5 ÷ 24 h
Step 3: Determine the insulin to carbohydrate ratio by one of the following formulas: • 450 ÷ total daily dose   • 6 × weight in kg ÷ total daily dose   • Total bolus dose divided by 3 meals   • Use existing carbohydrate ratio as before pump therapy
Step 4: Calculate the sensitivity/correction factor: • 1700 ÷ pump total daily dose
Step 5: Determine target blood glucose range
Step 6: Determine active insulin time[8,21,25]

entered into the calculator. The insulin pump calculates the bolus amount, which can be accepted, declined, or overridden. Finally, the calculator can ask if an extended or dual wave bolus is desired. Insulin pumps have an "insulin on board" feature that helps to prevent overtreatment of hyperglycemia. The insulin pump will subtract any insulin on board from a correction dose thereby, helping the user avoid subsequent hypoglycemia if to much insulin is given.

STARTING ON THE PUMP

There are many elements to keep in mind when helping a person select a pump. Does the person have certain accommodations that need to be addressed such as low vision, arthritis, neuropathy or extremes in ages such as children? Pump features to consider when selecting a brand include:

- Type of advanced features included,
- Watertight,
- Overall size,
- Ease of navigation screens and buttons,
- Screen visibility with backlight, good color contrast, use of icons, words, and abbreviations,
- Infusion site change reminders,
- Multiple languages,
- Communication with external glucose meter or continuous glucose monitor,
- Basal, boluses, and alarms history,
- Size of reservoir needed; length of tubing, length of catheter, and type of adhesive,
- Basal delivery rates; increments of basal rates, temporary or alternate basal rate options,
- Type of bolus offerings, sizes of bolus choices, remote bolus option, easy bolus, and calculator bolus,
- Safety issues, such as ability to stop bolus delivery,
- Lockout features for children,
- Warnings for no delivery, low battery, low reservoir, and so on,
- Option for a backup pump to be shipped, and
- Return and upgrade policy.[2]

Once a pump is selected, a diabetes educator or certified pump trainer will teach the user and their family how to use the pump. The medical provider will prescribe the initial dosages and calculations. (see **Table 3**). Fine tuning occurs slowly as the patient becomes familiar with the pump.

TROUBLESHOOTING

An insulin pump requires troubleshooting to avoid catastrophic problems. The user must be to ready for unexpected issues. Troubleshooting is one of the most important skills a pump wearer and their support system need to completely understand.

HYPERGLYCEMIA

One of the most frequent and possibly the most dangerous problems to occur with the pump is hyperglycemia. Because the insulin pump only contains rapid- or short-acting insulin, any disruption in insulin delivery can cause a rapid increase in BG. Emergency supplies must be carried at all times in case something happens to any part of the pump system. Supplies needed include new batteries, reservoir, infusion set, an insulin vial or pen, syringes or pen needles, alcohol wipes, adhesive, ketone strips, tape, glucose meter, strips, treatment for hypoglycemia, medical alert, list of pump settings, and medical team contact information. The pump manufacture number is on the back of the pump.

The American Association of Diabetes Educators (2017) offers a helpful troubleshooting teaching aid to assist in finding solutions to pump system related problems at https://www.diabeteseducator.org/docs/default-source/patient-resources/tip-sheets/insulin-infusion-sets/troubleshootingguide.pdf?sfvrsn=2.

Common causes of hyperglycemia in insulin pump wearers include the following.[4,16,26–28]

- Infusion set issues:
  - Kinked or dislodged tubing or cannula,
  - Air bubbles in tubing,
  - Leaking reservoir,
  - Infusion set coming loose, and
  - Prolonged disconnection (sports, sexual intimacy, swimming or bathing).
- Pump-related issues:
  - Batteries died,
  - Pump ran out of insulin,
  - Pump failure,
  - Pumps settings incorrectly set, and
  - Bolus not given or underbolused, or given late after food intake.
- Skin-related issues:
  - Insulin malabsorption from blood at site, lipohypertrophy, or scar tissue, and
  - Infection at infusion site.
- Metabolic issues:
  - Menstrual cycle,
  - Infection, illness, or injury,
  - New medications, especially steroids,
  - Recent hypoglycemia,
  - Change in eating patterns or food,
  - Stress,
  - Decreased physical activity, and
  - Change in sleeping cycles.
- Other issues
  - Glucometer errors and strip issues, and
  - Bad insulin

Once hyperglycemia is discovered, a treatment protocol needs to be initiated. The person must treat their diabetes first, then troubleshoot the pump second. The steps of the hyperglycemia protocol are as follows.

1. Treat the first BG above 250 mg/dL with a correction bolus via the pump.
2. Recheck BG in 1 hour. If the BG is improving, then no further action is necessary.
3. If the BG is not improving, give an insulin injection with a syringe or pen using the following formula: current BG – target BG ÷ correction factor.
4. Recheck the BG in 1 hour. If the BG is improving, change the infusion set with fresh insulin and a fresh injection site. If the BG is not improving, check ketones, take a correction dose using fresh insulin, and contact the prescriber. Do not continue using the insulin pump until the problem is identified.

HYPOGLYCEMIA

Hypoglycemia often occurs quickly and can be dangerous. When a low BG is experienced, there is a 46% chance of having another one the next day, 24% chance 2 days later, and 12% on the third day.[29] Common causes of hypoglycemia include:

- The basal, carbohydrate ratio, or correction factor too high,
- Inaccurate carbohydrate counting,
- Missed or delayed meals after bolusing,
- Insulin timing not matched to food intake,
- Drinking alcohol,
- Overriding the pump recommendations for treatment of hyperglycemia,
- Overriding the bolus calculator and choosing a higher dose,
- Exercise or increased activity,
- Hormonal changes, and
- A new infusion site that absorbs more quickly than previous sites.[2,16,26]

Treatment of hypoglycemia is as follows.

1. If the BG is 50 to 70 mg/dL, give 15 g of simple carbohydrate, and if the BG is less than 50 mg/dL, give 30 g by mouth if the patient can swallow.
2. Retest BG in 15 minutes and retreat if necessary.

Examples of 15 g of simple carbohydrate include:

- 1 tbsp honey,
- Glucose tablets or gel,
- 5 to 6 Lifesavers,
- 4 to 6 oz of regular soda, and
- 4 oz of juice.[26]

Administer glucagon or intravenous dextrose if the patient is unable to swallow carbohydrate. Glucagon comes in powder form in a kit that has a syringe of diluting fluid. The glucagon is diluted and can be injected subcutaneously, intravenously, or intramuscularly.[30,31]

SUMMARY

In summary, insulin pumps are a wonderful tool to help obtain tighter BG control and more flexibility. Just as health care providers become proficient with any type of technology, they should find that using a pump becomes less intimidating over time. There are plenty of online resources and pump trainers from the various pump manufacturers to help both users and medical providers to improve knowledge and skills.

REFERENCES

1. Heinemann L, Fleming GA, Petrie JR, et al. Insulin pump risks and benefits: a clinical appraisal of pump safety standards, adverse event reporting, and research needs. A Joint statement of the European Association for the Study of Diabetes and the American Diabetes Association Diabetes Technology Working Group. Diabetes Care 2015;38(4):716–22.
2. Bolderman KM. Putting your patients on the pump: initiation and maintenance guidelines. 2nd edition. Alexandria (VA): American Diabetes Association; 2013.
3. Walsh J, Roberts R. Pumping insulin, everything you need for success with an insulin pump. 3rd edition. San Diego (CA): Torres Pines Press; 2000.

4. Diabetes.co.uk.: the global diabetes community. Insulin Pumps. 2014. Available at: http://www.diabetes.co.uk/insulin/Insulin-pumps.html. Accessed April 14, 2017.

5. National Institutes of Health National Institute of Diabetes and Digestive and Kidney Diseases. DCCT and EDIC: the diabetes control and complication trial and followup study. In: SERVICES USDOHAH, editor. Bethesda (MD): National Diabetes Information Clearing House; 2008. Available at: https://www.niddk.nih.gov/about-niddk/research-areas/diabetes/dcct-edic-diabetes-control-complications-trial-follow-up-study/Documents/DCCT-EDIC_508.pdf. Accessed April 14, 2017.

6. Diabetes Control Complications Trial/Epidemiology of Diabetes Interventions Complications Study Research Group. Intensive diabetes treatment and cardiovascular disease in patients with type 1 diabetes. N Engl J Med 2005;353(25): 2643–53.

7. McCrea D. Management of the hospitalized diabetes patient with an insulin pump. Crit Care Nurs Clin North Am 2013;25:111–21.

8. Phlexteck's Diabetes Information Site. Insulin pump, they've come a long way! In: Wayne, editor. Phlexteck's Diabetes Information Site. vol 2017. ND. Available at: http://www.phlex.org/Diabetes/information-about-diabetes/insulin-pump2.html.

9. Pickup JC, Keen H, Parsons JA, et al. Continuous subcutaneous insulin infusion: an approach to achieving normoglycaemia. Br Med J 1978;1(6107):204–7.

10. Zorn M. When was the insulin pump invented. Vision Launch, be the change 2014. Available at: http://visionlaunch.com/when-was-the-insulin-pump-invented/. Accessed April 14, 2017.

11. Pickup J, Ly T, Nicholas J, et al. Insulin pumps. Diabetes Technol Ther 2015; 17(S1):S21–6.

12. Sattley M. The History of Diabetes. Diabetes Health 2015.

13. Lee S. History of pump technology. Medscape nurses education. ND. Available at: http://www.medscape.org/viewarticle/460365_2. Accessed April 14, 2017.

14. Zhang Y, Jones PL, Klonoff DC. Second insulin pump safety meeting: summary report. Journal of Diabetes Science and Technology 2010;4(2):488–93.

15. Rubin R. Insulin pumps in diabetes management. Todays Dietician, the magazine for nutrition professionals 2013;15(2):50.

16. Walsh J, Roberts R. Pumping insulin: everything for success on an insulin pump and CGM. 6th edition. San Diego (CA): Torrey Pines Press; 2017.

17. Graff MR, Rubin RR, Walker EA. How diabetes specialists treat their own diabetes: findings from a study of the AADE and ADA membership. Diabetes Educ 2000;26(3):460–7.

18. Scheiner G. Product guide: insulin pumps, find the right device for you. Diabetes Forcast 2016.

19. American Diabetes Association. Advantages of using an insulin pump. 2013. Available at: http://www.diabetes.org/living-with-diabetes/treatment-and-care/medication/insulin/advantages-of-using-an-insulin-pump.html?referrer=https://www.google.com/. Accessed May 23, 2017.

20. Grunberger G, Abelseth J, Bailey T, et al. Consensus statement by the American Association of Clinical Endocrinologists/American College of Endocrinology insulin pump management task force. Endocr Pract 2014;20(5):463–89.

21. Diabetes Care Community Website. Who is the best candidate for an insulin pump? What are your responsibilities? 2017. Available at: https://www.diabetescarecommunity.ca/living-well-with-diabetes-articles/8389/. Accessed May 23, 2017.

22. Schwartz S. Insulin pumps for type 2 diabetes: are you a candidate? Diabetes Daily 2016. Available at: https://www.diabetesdaily.com/blog/2014/08/insulin-pumps-for-type-2-diabetes/.

23. Skyler JS, Ponder S, Kruger DF, et al. Is there a place for insulin pump therapy in your practice. Clinical Diabetes 2007;25(2):50.

24. Bode BW. Pumping protocols, a guide to insulin pump therapy initiation. Medtronic Diabetes, Inc; 2013.

25. Walsh J, Roberts R. Insulin pump. Diabetes mall. 2017. Available at: http://www.diabetesnet.com/diabetes-technology/insulin-pumps. Accessed May 23, 2017.

26. Wolpert H. Smart pumping for people with diabetes. A practical approach to mastering the insulin pump. Alexandria (VA): American Diabetes Association; 2002.

27. American Association of Diabetes Educators Educator Tools. Insulin, infusion set troubleshooting guide. Chicago: American Association of Diabetes Educators; 2017.

28. Medtronic Diabetes. The basics of insulin pump therapy. Northridge (CA): Medtronic Minimed, Inc.; 2010.

29. Cox D, Gonder-Federick L, Polonsky W, et al. Recent hypoglycemia influences the probability of subsequent hypoglycemia in type 1 patients. Paper presented at: American Diabetes Association Conference. Las Vegas, NV, June 12-15, 1993.

30. Haymond MW, Schreiner B. Mini-dose glucagon rescue for hypoglycemia in children with type 1 diabetes. Diabetes Care 2001;24(4):643–5.

31. Flynn M. Diabetes disaster averted #41: glucagon mini-dosing- a valuable tool. Diabetes in Control: News and information for medical professionals 2011.

Hypoglycemia in Diabetes

Marjorie R. Ortiz, RN, MSN, AGPCNP-BC

KEYWORDS

- Hypoglycemia • Diabetes • Hypoglycemia unawareness • Patient education

KEY POINTS

- Hypoglycemia is a limiting factor in achieving glucose control in patients with diabetes.
- Hypoglycemia is the result of increased insulin levels or decreased counterregulation in patients with diabetes.
- Recurrent hypoglycemia can cause autonomic failure and increased risk of hypoglycemia unawareness.
- Patient education and prevention strategies should be implemented between the patient and provider to recognize, manage, and prevent hypoglycemia.

INTRODUCTION

Hypoglycemia is a major limiting factor in achieving glycemic control in patients with diabetes. The American Diabetes Association recommends an HgA1C goal of less than 7% in most patients, and the American Association of Clinical Endocrinologists recommends an HgA1C less than 6.5%, if achievable without significant hypoglycemia.[1,2] Landmark studies, such as the Diabetes Control and Complications Trial and the United Kingdom Prospective Diabetes Trial have clearly shown that tight glycemic control can prevent or delay the development of microvascular complications, such as retinopathy, nephropaty, and neuropathy, in type 1 and type 2 diabetes, but with aggressive glycemic targets comes an increase of hypoglycemia risk.[3] Higher glycemic targets may be more appropriate in patients with recurring hypoglycemia, limited life span, or multiple comorbidities, and goals should be individualized per patient.[2] Balancing strict glucose control to prevent microvascular and avoidance of hypoglycemia can become a challenge for both providers and patients.

Hypoglycemia incidence in diabetes is often underestimated and underreported, especially mild or asymptomatic episodes. Hypoglycemia occurs more often in patients with type 1 diabetes, with an estimated 1 to 2 symptomatic episodes per week, and 1 episode of severe hypoglycemia per year.[4] The incidence of

Disclosure Statement: The author has nothing to disclose.
Department of Endocrine Neoplasia and Hormonal Disorders, MD Anderson Cancer Center, 1515 Holcombe Boulevard, Houston, TX 77030, USA
E-mail address: MOrtiz2@MDAnderson.org

hypoglycemia in type 2 diabetes is much lower than in patients with type 1 diabetes, but patients with longstanding type 2 diabetes on insulin therapy have comparable hypoglycemia rates to patients with type 1 diabetes.[5] Repeated hypoglycemia can impair the body's defenses against hypoglycemia, leading to recurrent and more severe episodes, and can be fatal. Hypoglycemia has been reported to cause 4% to 10% of deaths in patients with type 1 diabetes.[6]

Hypoglycemia can cause short term and long term problems. Symptoms of hypoglycemia are unpleasant, and can disrupt daily functions. If hypoglycemia occurs while driving, motor vehicle accidents can occur, causing injury to the patient and others. Hypoglycemia can decrease work performance, interfering with daily job requirements. It can cause falls, leading to injury. If severe enough, it can cause seizures and death.[4] Repeated hypoglycemia can cause loss of counterregulatory protective effects and hypoglycemia unawareness. Patients with recurrent hypoglycemia report higher fear of hypoglycemia leading to missed medication doses. Overtreatment of hypoglycemia, leading to overall worsening of glycemic control.[7]

Hypoglycemia has cardiovascular effects. Physiologically, it can increase cardiac contractility, cause electrocardiogram changes, and increase the workload of the heart.[4,8] Severe hypoglycemia has been associated with prolonging the QT interval. Death from hypoglycemia is thought to be caused by cardiac arrhythmias. The Action to Control Cardiovascular Risk in Diabetes (ACCORD) trial, which studied effects of intensive versus standard glucose control on cardiovascular events, was stopped prematurely due to increased mortality in the patients treated intensively. Hypoglycemia was significantly higher in the intensively treated group.[9]

Additionally, hypoglycemia can lead to increased emergency room admissions and health care costs[10,11] The Centers for Disease Control and Prevention estimated the amount of emergency room visits secondary to hypoglycemia in patients with diabetes to average 300,000 visits per year between 2006 and 2009.[12]

It is important for health care providers to understand this often-overlooked complication of diabetes management, to know which medications cause hypoglycemia, recognize which patients are at risk, and implement strategies to prevent future episodes of hypoglycemia to ensure the safety of patients. Patient education is key in the prevention and avoidance of hypoglycemia.

HYPOGLYCEMIA: DEFINITION

Hypoglycemia is defined as any glucose value low enough to harm a patient. Although no definite glucose value has been assigned to define hypoglycemia, as patients with diabetes may have differing symptoms at various glucose levels, a glucose value less than 70 mg/dL should alert a patient or provider of possible impending hypoglycemia.[6] The American Diabetes Association Workgroup on Hypoglycemia defines hypoglycemia in the following ways:

1. Severe hypoglycemia: an episode requiring third-party assistance for treatment of hypoglycemia, either with administration of carbohydrate, glucagon, or other forms of glucose.
2. Documented symptomatic hypoglycemia: an episode in which the patient experiences symptoms of hypoglycemia, and glucose measured at the time of symptoms is less than 70 mg/dL.
3. Asymptomatic hypoglycemia: an episode of glucose less than 70 mg/dL without any symptoms of hypoglycemia.
4. Probable symptomatic hypoglycemia: an episode of symptoms indicating hypoglycemia, but without documentation of glucose less than 70 mg/dL.

5. Pseudo-hypoglycemia: an episode in which the patient reports symptoms of hypo-glycemia, but glucose is higher than 70 mg/dL.[6] Some patients with poor glucose control may experience symptoms of hypoglycemia at normal glucose values.

GLUCOSE REGULATION

Glucose provides fuel for energy, particularly the brain. The brain requires a contin-uous influx of glucose to function properly. Glucose is supplied exogenously, through ingested food, or endogenously, mostly stored in the liver in the form of glycogen. The kidneys play a role in glucose homeostasis, providing glucose through gluconeogen-esis, and reabsorption of glucose through the proximal tubule. Normally, when plasma glucose levels fall, the body goes through a series of changes to increase glucose levels and maintain homeostasis. **Fig. 1** illustrates these hormonal changes as glucose levels decrease. The first change, which occurs at glucose levels between 80 and 85 mg/dL is a decrease in insulin secretion from the pancreas. This is the first line of defense against hypoglycemia. This decrease in insulin increases hepatic and renal glucose production to increase overall glucose levels. The second line of defense oc-curs as glucose levels reach 65 to 70 mg/dL. At these glucose levels, glucagon is secreted from the pancreatic alpha cells into the hepatic portal vein. Glucagon stim-ulates hepatic glucose production through glycogenolysis. The third line of defense is release of epinephrine, cortisol, and growth hormone, which also occurs at glucose levels in the range of 65 to 70 mg/dL. Epinephrine raises glucose levels through many mechanisms. It stimulates hepatic glycogenolysis and renal gluconeogenesis, sup-presses insulin secretion from the pancreas, and increases glycolysis and lipolysis in muscle and fat. As glucose levels fall farther below 60 mg/dL, neuroglycopenic symptoms occur, prompting the patient to treat hypoglycemia by ingesting

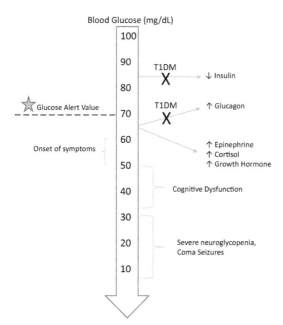

Fig. 1. Counterregulatory response to hypoglycemia. Up arrows indicate increasing. Down arrows indicate decreasing.

carbohydrate.[13] As glucose lowers below 50 mg/dL, cognition is altered. Prolonged very low glucose levels can cause brain death.[14]

In type 1 diabetes, this feedback mechanism is impaired. Patients with type 1 diabetes are insulin deficient, meaning the pancreatic beta cells do not produce insulin. These patients require exogenous subcutaneous insulin injections. When glucose levels drop, circulating insulin levels in patients with type 1 diabetes do not decrease as they would in patients with intact pancreatic function. These patients are also glucagon deficient. This results in loss of both the first and second lines of defense against hypoglycemia, predisposing these patients to more frequent and severe hypoglycemia. Patients with Type 1 diabetes are critically dependent on the third line of defense to combat hypoglycemia.[15]

RISK FACTORS FOR HYPOGLYCEMIA

In patients with diabetes, hypoglycemia is caused by increased circulating insulin levels and/or decreased defenses against hypoglycemia. Medications that increase insulin levels include injectable insulin, sulfonylureas, or meglitinides. Although other classes of medications, such as biguanides, thiazolidinediones, glucagonlike peptide 1 (GLP-1) agonists, alpha-glucosidase inhibitors, and dipeptidyl peptidase-4 (DPP-IV) inhibitors do not cause hypoglycemia directly, combinations of these agents with higher risk hypoglycemic agents, such as insulin, sulfonylureas, and metiglinides, can increase the risk of low blood sugars. Unlike GLP-1 receptor agonists and DPP-IV inhibitors, which stimulate pancreatic insulin secretion in response to hyperglycemia, sulfonylureas stimulate insulin release regardless of glucose level.

Intensive insulin regimens and lower HgA1C targets also place patients at risk of hypoglycemia.[15] There are many different insulins on the US market today. The type and doses of insulin prescribed are individualized per patient, and are dependent on insurance preference, amount of injections per day, motivation of the patient, willingness of the patient to inject insulin, degree of hyperglycemia, among others. Any patient who injects insulin is at risk of hypoglycemia.

Patients taking basal and bolus insulin (long-acting and rapid-acting insulins) require intensive glucose monitoring and multiple doses of insulin per day. The goal of basal bolus is to mimic physiologic insulin production. The pancreas secretes or inhibits insulin in response to rising or falling glucose levels. Basal insulin is used to control liver glucose output, whereas bolus or mealtime insulin is used to control hyperglycemia from food intake. Prolonged fasting status, skipped meals, delayed meals, unfinished meals, or incorrect timing of insulin doses in relation to food can cause hypoglycemia. Patients who take premixed insulin, which contains both intermediate and rapid-acting insulin in one injection, are at higher risk of developing hypoglycemia if meals are skipped or inconsistent.[16]

Hypoglycemia frequently occurs overnight. It is the longest fasting period of the day, and insulin sensitivity increases between 1 AM and 3 AM. Patients may be unable to recognize hypoglycemia symptoms during sleep. Nocturnal hypoglycemia may cause rebound hyperglycemia on awakening.[17] Insulin sensitivity is also increased during exercise and after weight loss. Glucose needs increase during periods of activity, and glycogen stores are rapidly used.[17] Low blood sugars can occur while exercising, or hours after exercise has ended.

Patients with altered mental status, or in situations in which mentation is impaired also risk hypoglycemia. Patients with altered mental status may not be able to acknowledge or verbalize the symptoms, and may not be able to ask for help or treat themselves. Alcohol and illicit substances can block perception of symptoms, inhibiting early recognition and treatment of symptoms.[15] Alcohol also impairs gluconeogenesis.

Renal, hepatic, or adrenal dysfunction can alter the response to hypoglycemia. In patients with renal dysfunction, medication clearance is slowed, prolonging the effects of medications such as insulin, sulfonylureas, and metiglinides. Patients with hepatic impairment may not be able to respond to hypoglycemia due to decreased glycogen stores. Patients with adrenal insufficiency are unable to respond to hypoglycemia because of impaired counterregulatory hormones.

Elderly patients have a higher risk of hypoglycemia. Factors that place this population at risk include decreased clearance of medication, impaired cognition, and inability to recognize signs and symptoms of hypoglycemia. Hypoglycemia can lead to increased falls and injury in this population. Hospital admissions for hypoglycemia is higher in this population than in younger patients.[18] Very young patients are also at risk for similar reasons, such as inability to verbalize symptoms and inability to treat themselves when hypoglycemic.

Postponing treatment of a mild hypoglycemic episode can place patients at risk for developing more severe hypoglycemia in the future.[15]

Health care providers should be aware of these risk factors for hypoglycemia, and be cautious when prescribing or administering certain medications to these particular patients. **Box 1** shows a list of these risk factors.

SYMPTOMS

Symptoms of hypoglycemia can vary among patients. The threshold of symptomatic hypoglycemia is lower in patients with well-controlled diabetes, and higher in patients with poorly controlled diabetes.[19] Symptoms are divided into 2 categories: neuroglycopenic or autonomic. Neuroglycopenic symptoms are the direct result of lack of

---

Box 1
Risk factors for hypoglycemia

- Medications: insulin, sulfonylureas, metiglinides
- Type 1 diabetes or longstanding type 2 diabetes
- Longer duration of diabetes diagnosis
- Low A1C
- Age: elderly or very young
- Exercise
- Prolonged fasting
- Mismatched dose or timing of insulin with food
- Renal or hepatic dysfunction
- Sleep
- Alcohol
- Exercise
- Weight loss
- Adrenal insufficiency
- Prior hypoglycemia/recurrent hypoglycemia

glucose to the brain, and includes symptoms such as confusion, weakness, fatigue, slurred speech, hunger, and more severe symptoms such as coma and death. Autonomic symptoms include pallor, anxiety, palpitations, numbness/tingling, tremors, and diaphoresis.[17] With mild symptoms, patients are usually able to treat themselves. More severe symptoms, including altered mental status, unconsciousness, seizures, and coma require third-party assistance. The degree of symptoms and threshold of which patients experience symptoms depend on their overall glucose control, and frequency of hypoglycemia. Patients with an elevated HgA1C may experience hypoglycemia symptoms at a normal glucose level due to hyperglycemia at baseline. Patients with low HgA1C levels or frequent hypoglycemia may not experience hypoglycemic symptoms until glucose reaches a lower level. The higher frequency of hypoglycemic episodes, the lower the threshold becomes for symptoms to occur. These patients are at higher risk for developing hypoglycemic unawareness.

HYPOGLYCEMIA UNAWARENESS

Recurrent episodes of hypoglycemia can inhibit a patient's defense mechanisms against hypoglycemia. With each occurrence of hypoglycemia, glucose levels need become even lower to elicit symptoms.[15] Patients who are asymptomatic at glucose levels lower than 55 mg/dL should notify their providers for evaluation of hypoglycemia unawareness.

Hypoglycemia-associated autonomic failure (HAAF) is a combination of ineffective glucose counterregulatory mechanisms and compromised awareness of hypoglycemia. It is caused by recent and recurrent hypoglycemia. Risk factors for HAAF include duration of diabetes, absence of endogenous insulin production, recent and frequent hypoglycemia, and hypoglycemia unawareness. Hypoglycemia unawareness can be reversed by allowing glucose levels to run above target to reset the internal alarm clock to alert when glucose levels are falling. By avoiding hypoglycemia for 2 to 3 weeks, hypoglycemia awareness can be reestablished.

HYPOGLYCEMIA TREATMENT

If hypoglycemia is suspected, glucose should be checked to confirm. If equipment is not available at the time, the patient or caregiver should assume that the glucose level is low and treat the symptoms. With mild hypoglycemia in patients who are awake and able to take liquids by mouth, 15 to 20 g of fast-acting carbohydrates should be ingested at the time of hypoglycemia symptoms. Foods with high fat or protein content are not good treatments for hypoglycemia, because the other macronutrients can slow the absorption of glucose. **Box 2** lists options for treatment of hypoglycemia.

It is important to not overtreat the hypoglycemia. Ingesting higher amounts of glucose or carbohydrates can lead to overcorrection and subsequent hyperglycemia. Glucose should be rechecked 15 minutes after the initial intervention. If the patient remains hypoglycemic, this process should be repeated until glucose is above 70 mg/dL. After glucose is above 70 mg/dL, the patient should have a meal or snack to prevent hypoglycemia from recurring.[2]

In severe hypoglycemia, when the patient requires third-party assistance, the patient should not be given oral carbohydrate, as this can cause aspiration if the patient has altered mental status and is unable to swallow. These patients should be given glucagon intramuscularly or dextrose intravenously. Glucagon requires a prescription and education on its use. Glucagon 1 mg is the dose indicated for most adults. If a patient has intravenous access, 10 to 25 g 50% dextrose should be given. Again, glucose should be repeated every 15 minutes until glucose is higher than 70 mg/dL.

Box 2
Examples of 15 to 20 g of fast-acting carbohydrate

- 4 glucose tablets
- 4 ounces of fruit juice
- 5 to 6 ounces of regular soda (nondiet)
- 7 to 8 gummy bears or regular life savers
- 1 tablespoon of sugar or jelly
- 1 glucose gel pack
- 10 to 15 jelly beans
- 15 Skittles
- 1 tablespoon of honey
- 1 cup low-fat milk
- 1 tablespoon table sugar

Intravenous dextrose is preferred to glucagon, if there is access to medical personnel and equipment.[2]

HYPOGLYCEMIA: PATIENT EDUCATION, EVALUATION, AND PREVENTION
Patient Education

Education should start at the first visit between the patient and the provider. If resources are available, involving a diabetes educator, nursing staff, and dietician is beneficial to the patient. First and foremost, patients should be taught self-monitoring of blood glucose (SMBG). The frequency of SMBG is dependent on which medications the patient is prescribed. If low-risk hypoglycemic agents are prescribed, the patient may be asked by the provider to check glucose levels only occasionally. However, if a patient is started on high-risk hypoglycemic agents, or insulin injections, glucose will need to be checked more frequently. Patients should be encouraged to bring their glucometer or log book to each visit, to be reviewed by the provider. HgA1C should not be a sole indicator of glycemic control in patients who have frequent hypoglycemia, as the result can be skewed if there are wide fluctuations in blood sugars. Patients with frequent hypoglycemia may have an acceptable, or even low HgA1C value.

When hypoglycemic agents are prescribed, patients should be educated about the hypoglycemic risk, as well as the onset, peak, and duration of the medication. In patients who have frequent hypoglycemia, or if the risk of hypoglycemia outweighs the benefit of better glucose control, the provider should consider switching to a class of medication with less hypoglycemic risk. Timing of the medication in relation to food or glucose level, as well as risk of skipping meals, prolonged fasting, and alcohol should be included in the patient education.[20] Other factors that contribute to hypoglycemia, such as exercise, weight loss, and nocturnal hypoglycemia, also should be discussed. If necessary, SMBG should be done before exercise, sleep, and driving.

Patients should be educated about the signs, symptoms, and treatment of hypoglycemia. Patients should be alerted if glucose is less than 70 mg/dL, even if no symptoms are present. Patients at risk for hypoglycemia should carry a form of carbohydrate with them at all times should symptoms occur. Treatment of glucose less than 70 mg/dL and not delaying treatment can prevent progression to more severe hypoglycemia.[20]

It is important for patients to be educated on which foods raise blood glucose levels. For patients who take mealtime insulin, it is important to educate on the importance of a consistent carbohydrate diet. If the patient eats less carbohydrate than usual, but takes the same amount of insulin, there is potential for hypoglycemia after that meal. Patients with type 1 diabetes should be taught to count carbohydrates to more effectively dose mealtime insulin. Patients taking premixed insulin also should be educated on the importance of consistent meals, because the insulin has both longer-acting and shorter-acting insulin in one injection. Patients who skip meals frequently are at higher risk of hypoglycemia if taking premixed insulin.

Evaluation of Hypoglycemia

In subsequent visits with the provider, assessment of hypoglycemia during each visit is needed to identify if the problem exists. Evaluation of hypoglycemia frequency, severity, and presence of hypoglycemia awareness should be assessed at each visit. Examples of questions to ask the patient include the following:

- Do you check your blood sugar? How often? What are the usual values?
- Do you ever have any blood sugars less than 70 mg/dL?
  - If yes, when does this usually occur? How often does this occur?
  - Do you have any symptoms at those times?
  - What symptoms do you experience?
  - If no, do you ever have any signs of hypoglycemia, such as diaphoresis, palpitations, or anxiety?
- What do you do when you have a blood sugar less than 70 mg/dL, or when you experience symptoms of low blood sugars?
- How low does your blood sugar have to be for you to feel symptoms?
- Have you ever needed help from someone else to treat a low blood sugar?
- Have you ever been hospitalized or had to call for emergency assistance due to low blood sugar?

Once hypoglycemia is identified, risk factors and contributing factors should be assessed, and if needed, modification in the medication regimen should be made. The goal is to limit the frequency and duration of hypoglycemia without having subsequent hyperglycemia and worsening glucose control. Identifying certain situations that trigger hypoglycemia is important in prevention of future episodes. Examples of questions to ask the patient include the following:

- Does hypoglycemia happen at any particular time of day?
- Does hypoglycemia occur during any specific activities?
- How does hypoglycemia affect your daily life?
- Do you ever miss medication/insulin doses for fear of hypoglycemia, or to prevent hypoglycemia?

Interventions and Prevention Strategies

Once the cause of hypoglycemia is identified, medication changes may need to be made by the provider. For suspected nocturnal hypoglycemia, the following interventions can be implemented: glucose monitoring before bedtime, on awakening, and occasionally between 1 and 3 AM. The provider may adjust the pre-bedtime doses of medication, or ask the patient to have a snack before bedtime, to prevent further nocturnal hypoglycemia.

If hypoglycemia occurs during exercise, patients should be encouraged to monitor their glucose levels before and after exercise, and if needed, either ingest more carbohydrate before exercise, or modify their medication doses before exercise. Teaching the patient how to modify his or her insulin doses according to hypoglycemia triggering situations also can prevent future hypoglycemia. These adjustments should be done at the instruction and help of a diabetes provider.

In some patients with problematic hypoglycemia already taking multiple-dose insulin, switching therapy to an insulin pump and continuous glucose monitors may be considered.[20] Insulin pumps can provide multiple rates of insulin administration throughout the day, allowing more insulin administration in times of increased insulin needs, and less insulin administration at times when insulin sensitivity is increased.[6] Certain insulin pumps have a basal suspend setting, whereby insulin delivery is suspended when the continuous glucose monitor senses hypoglycemia.

Continuous glucose monitors (CGMs) are devices that measure interstitial glucose levels at frequent intervals (every 1–5 minutes). CGMs display the interstitial glucose levels, as well as the direction and rate of change of glucose. These devices are able to alarm not only at certain glucose values, but at rate of decrease of the glucose values, allowing the patient to be notified before hypoglycemia occurs. CGMs allow providers to determine trends in glucose values. Patients who consistently wear CGMs reported less worry about hypoglycemia, which may increase quality of life.[21] Use of CGMs also can reduce severe hypoglycemia in patients with hypoglycemia unawareness.[20]

In patients with hypoglycemia unawareness, involving family or support systems in the care of the patient becomes very important. The patient and family members should be taught how to use glucagon, and a prescription should be written for glucagon by the provider. Patients with hypoglycemia unawareness should be encouraged to monitor glucose more frequently, at least before each meal and at bedtime, and occasionally during the night, to assess for nocturnal hypoglycemia.

SUMMARY

Hypoglycemia is a common problem in patients with diabetes, often preventing patients from achieving optimal glucose control. Hypoglycemia can cause anxiety, lead to noncompliance with medication regimens, and decrease quality of life. Severe cases can cause cardiac rhythm abnormalities and can be fatal. Patient and caregiver/family education on SMBG, risk factors for developing hypoglycemia, medication education, and prevention strategies are beneficial in the prevention of developing hypoglycemia. Avoidance of hypoglycemia can help in achieving optimal glucose control in patients with diabetes.

REFERENCES

1. Handelsman Y, Bloomgarden ZT, Grunberger G, et al. American Association of Clinical Endocrinologists and American College of Endocrinology–clinical practice guidelines for developing a diabetes mellitus comprehensive care plan–2015. Endocr Pract 2015;21(s1):1–87.

2. Marathe PH, Gao HX, Close KL. American Diabetes Association standards of medical care in diabetes 2017. J Diabetes 2017;9(4):320–4.

3. Nathan DM, Group DER. The diabetes control and complications trial/epidemiology of diabetes interventions and complications study at 30 years: overview. Diabetes Care 2014;37(1):9–16.

4. Frier BM. Hypoglycaemia in diabetes mellitus: epidemiology and clinical implications. Nat Rev Endocrinol 2014;10(12):711–22.

5. UK Hypoglycaemia Study Group. Risk of hypoglycaemia in types 1 and 2 diabetes: effects of treatment modalities and their duration. Diabetologia 2007; 50(6):1140–7.

6. Seaquist ER, Anderson J, Childs B, et al. Hypoglycemia and diabetes: a report of a workgroup of the American Diabetes Association and the Endocrine Society. Diabetes Care 2013;36(5):1384–95.

7. McCoy R, Van Houten H, Ziegenfuss J, et al. Self-report of hypoglycemia and health-related quality of life in patients with type 1 and type 2 diabetes. Endocr Pract 2013;19(5):792–9.

8. Frier BM, Schernthaner G, Heller SR. Hypoglycemia and cardiovascular risks. Diabetes Care 2011;34(Supplement 2):S132–7.

9. ACCORD Study Group, Buse JB, Bigger JT, et al. Action to control cardiovascular risk in diabetes (ACCORD) trial: design and methods. Am J Cardiol 2007;99(12): S21–33.

10. Foos V, Varol N, Curtis BH, et al. Economic impact of severe and non-severe hypoglycemia in patients with Type 1 and Type 2 diabetes in the United States. J Med Econ 2015;18(6):420–32.

11. Quilliam BJ, Simeone JC, Ozbay AB, et al. The incidence and costs of hypoglycemia in type 2 diabetes. Am J Manag Care 2011;17(10):673–80.

12. Centers for Disease Control and Prevention. National diabetes statistics report: estimates of diabetes and its burden in the United States, 2014. 2014. Available at: http://www.cdc.gov/diabetes/data/statistics/2014statisticsreport.html. Accessed February 1, 2017.

13. Cryer P. Hypoglycemia in diabetes: pathophysiology, prevalence, and prevention. Alexandria (VA): American Diabetes Association; 2016.

14. Cryer PE. Hypoglycemia, functional brain failure, and brain death. J Clin Invest 2007;117(4):868–70.

15. Kaufman FR. Medical management of type 1 diabetes. Alexandria (VA): American Diabetes Association; 2012.

16. Unger J. Uncovering undetected hypoglycemic events. Diabetes Metab Syndr Obes 2012;5:57–74.

17. Fonseca VA. Clinical diabetes: translating research into practice. Philadelphia: Elsevier; 2006.

18. Lipska KJ, Ross JS, Wang Y, et al. National trends in US hospital admissions for hyperglycemia and hypoglycemia among Medicare beneficiaries, 1999 to 2011. JAMA Intern Med 2014;174(7):1116–24.

19. International Hypoglycaemia Study Group. Minimizing hypoglycemia in diabetes. Diabetes Care 2015;38(8):1583–91.

20. Choudhary P, Rickels MR, Senior PA, et al. Evidence-informed clinical practice recommendations for treatment of type 1 diabetes complicated by problematic hypoglycemia. Diabetes Care 2015;38(6):1016–29.

21. Chamberlain JJ, Dopita D, Gilgen E, et al. Impact of frequent and persistent use of continuous glucose monitoring (CGM) on hypoglycemia fear, frequency of emergency medical treatment, and SMBG frequency after one year. J Diabetes Sci Technol 2016;10(2):383–8.

Management Strategies for Patients with Diabetic Kidney Disease and Chronic Kidney Disease in Diabetes

Jessica K. Yakush Williams, MSPAS, PA-C

KEYWORDS

- Diabetes mellitus • Diabetic kidney disease (DKD) • Chronic kidney disease (CKD)
- Microvascular complications of diabetes

KEY POINTS

- Chronic kidney disease (CKD) is a common microvascular complication of diabetes mellitus.
- Diabetic kidney disease (DKD) is defined as CKD caused by diabetes mellitus, which is the leading cause of kidney failure in the United States.
- Albuminuria and estimated glomerular filtration rate are biomarkers used to monitor development and progression of DKD.
- Management strategies for DKD and CKD are complex and multifaceted, including lifestyle management and pharmacologic management.
- The number of pharmacologic agents available for use in DKD has grown tremendously, and further research continues to evaluate potential new biomarkers for monitoring DKD and potential new therapies that may slow progression of DKD.

INTRODUCTION

Diabetes mellitus (to be referred to as diabetes in text, DM in tables) is a chronic condition that leads to high medical costs, increased risks for developing life-altering and life-threatening complications, and contributes to significant morbidity and mortality in patients afflicted with this disease. In 2007, incidence rates for diabetes were 7.8 cases per 1000 people and projections were showing an expected increase in prevalence of 33% by 2050.[1] In 2012, total costs in the United States due to diabetes were in excess of $245 billion with the expectation that costs will continue to rise.[2] Patients with diabetes are at risk for developing an array of microvascular and macrovascular

Disclosure Statement: There are no conflicts of interest or disclosures to report.
Department of Endocrine Neoplasia and Hormonal Disorders, University of Texas MD Anderson Cancer Center, 1515 Holcombe Boulevard, Houston, TX 77030, USA
E-mail address: jkwilliams1@mdanderson.org

Nurs Clin N Am 52 (2017) 575–587
http://dx.doi.org/10.1016/j.cnur.2017.07.007
nursing.theclinics.com

complications. Kidney disease is one of the most common microvascular complications of diabetes and has a significant impact on a patient's health care and potentially his or her quality of life. Diabetes is and has been the leading cause of kidney failure in the United States leading many individuals to come to rely on dialysis or the need for a kidney transplant.[3]

Between 2008 and 2012, the incidence of diabetic patients beginning treatment for end-stage renal disease (ESRD) rose by approximately 1000 patients.[2,3] More concerning, however, is that the prevalence of those already in treatment for ESRD increased by nearly 30,000 individuals over the course of 4 years (**Table 1**).[2,3] That is a nearly 14% increase in the prevalence of ESRD, which is a debilitating and life-threatening condition for those affected. It is for this reason that close attention must be paid to this important and life-altering complication of diabetes.

DEFINITION AND RISK FACTORS

Diabetic kidney disease (DKD), defined as chronic kidney disease (CKD) due to diabetes, occurs in approximately 20% to 40% of diabetic patients.[4] Not only does this make it a common complication, but it is also important to reiterate that diabetes mellitus remains the leading cause of ESRD in the United States.[4,5] Apart from having diabetes, there are multiple other risk factors that may help to predict who may develop DKD and to what severity (**Table 2**). Some of these include intrinsic factors, which are risk factors that cannot be altered. For example, differences in rates of DKD are seen across ethnic lines: African American, Hispanic, and Native American individuals continue to have higher incidences rates of development of ESRD.[4] Because these factors are not changeable, management targets those factors that are modifiable, such as glycemic control, blood pressure (BP), and lipid management. Both estimated glomerular filtration rate (eGFR) and albuminuria are the most useful biomarkers currently available for monitoring for progression of kidney disease. Glycemic control, BP, and dyslipidemia management all play a role in preventing the advancement of kidney disease when properly addressed.[6]

PATHOPHYSIOLOGY OF DIABETIC KIDNEY DISEASE

The pathophysiology of DKD is exceedingly complex. In brief, all anatomic components of the kidney are involved in the development and progression of DKD. The

Table 1
Incidence and prevalence of ESRD in DM patients from 2008 to 2012

	No. of Patients with DM Beginning Treatment for ESRD	No. of Patients with DM Living on Dialysis or with Kidney Transplant
2008	48,000	202,000
2012	49,000	229,000

Abbreviations: DM, diabetes mellitus; ESRD, end-stage renal disease.
Data from Centers for Disease Control and Prevention. National diabetes statistics report: estimates of diabetes and its burden in the United States, 2014. Atlanta (GA): US Department of Health and Human Services; 2014. p. 1-12; and Centers for Disease Control and Prevention. National diabetes fact sheet: national estimates and general information on diabetes and prediabetes in the United States, 2011. Atlanta (GA): US Department of Health and Human Services, Centers for Disease Control and Prevention; 2011. p. 1-12.

Table 2
Risk factors associated with development of diabetic kidney disease

Modifiable Risk Factors	Intrinsic Risk Factors
Hyperglycemia	Age
Hypertension	Sex
Albuminuria	Ethnicity
Dyslipidemia	Family history
Smoking	Duration of diabetes

Data from MacIsaac RJ, Ekinci EI, Jerums G. Markers of and risk factors for the development and progression of diabetic kidney disease. Am J Kidney Dis 2014;63(2, Supplement 2):S39–62.

changes that occur in these anatomic structures with prolonged exposure to hyperglycemia result in albuminuria, reduced eGFR, elevation in arterial BP, and fluid retention, all of which are mediated by several pathways.[7] The major players in these pathways are the renin-angiotensin-aldosterone system (RAAS), profibrotic and inflammatory cytokines, and various signaling kinases.[7] The RAAS pathway has been a prime target for medical management of both hypertension and CKD due to the available pharmaceutical agents that inhibit this pathway, which include angiotensin-converting-enzyme (ACE) inhibitors and angiotensin-receptor-blockers (ARBs). It is important to keep in mind there are multiple other intricate pathways that further contribute to the development of DKD which are not yet fully understood, and could potentially lead to future pharmacologic advancements as ongoing studies continue to reveal more data.

DIAGNOSIS AND MONITORING

The diagnosis of DKD is made by assessment of eGFR and urine albumin excretion (albuminuria) which is measured as the urine albumin-to-creatinine ratio.

- DKD is characterized by eGFR of less than 60 mL/min/1.73 m^2 and albuminuria greater than 30 mg/g.[4]
- DKD develops approximately 10 years after development of diabetes, although in type 2 diabetes many patients may already have DKD at the time of diagnosis.[5]
- Screening for changes in eGFR and albuminuria should be done at least once a year in all patients with type 2 diabetes, including at the time of diagnosis, whereas screening should begin 5 years after diagnosis in those with type 1 diabetes.[5]

Screening for albuminuria is typically done by spot urinary albumin-to-creatinine ratio or by timed 24-hour urine collections; however, the latter is more cumbersome for patients. Of note, if an elevated result is obtained, it should be repeated 2 to 3 times within a 3-month to 6-month period to truly confirm the presence of albuminuria, because a single elevated reading may not be reliable.[5] For example, recent exercise, infection, fever, congestive heart failure, hyperglycemia, menstruation, or marked hypertension can elevate the degree of albuminuria leading to the possibility of false positive readings. Serum creatinine and potassium also should be monitored annually in addition to albuminuria and eGFR as additional markers of disease progression.[5] Screening and monitoring recommendations are summarized in **Table 3**.

It should be noted that not all diabetic patients with CKD have DKD, as CKD can arise from other pathologies independent of diabetes. The following are clinical

Table 3	
Recommended monitoring for CKD in DM	
Type 1 diabetes	Monitoring for DKD to begin 5 y after diagnosis
Type 2 diabetes	Monitoring should begin at the time of diagnosis
eGFR (mL/min/1.73m²)	*Recommendation*
Any eGFR	• Annual screening of urine albumin-creatinine ratio, serum creatinine, and potassium
45–60	• Review medications and consider dose adjustment as indicated • Monitor eGFR every 6 mo • Monitor for electrolyte abnormalities, anemia, vitamin D status, calcium, phosphorus, and parathyroid hormone annually • Vaccinate against hepatitis B virus • Consider bone density testing • Refer to nutritionist
30–44	• Review medications and consider dose adjustment as indicated • Monitor eGFR every 3 mo • Monitor for electrolyte abnormalities, anemia, calcium, phosphorus and parathyroid hormone every 3–6 mo
<30	• Refer to a nephrologist

Abbreviations: CKD, chronic kidney disease; DKD, diabetic kidney disease; DM, diabetes mellitus; eGFR, estimated glomerular filtration rate.

Data from Marathe PH, Gao HX, Close KL. American Diabetes Association standards of medical care in diabetes 2017. J Diabetes 2017;9(4):320–4.

indicators that should prompt the medical provider to consider other etiologies of CKD, even in diabetic patients:

- Absence of diabetic retinopathy (especially in type 1 diabetes)
- Rapidly decreasing eGFR
- Nephrotic syndrome (rapidly increasing proteinuria)
- Refractory hypertension
- Active urinary sediment
- Other systemic disease
- Greater than 30% reduction in eGFR within 2 to 3 months after starting ACE inhibitor or ARB
- Abnormal findings on renal ultrasound[4,5,8]

If at any time it is suspected that the patient's CKD is due to a reason other than diabetes, the patient should be referred to a nephrologist for further evaluation.

MANAGEMENT GOALS AND STRATEGIES
Nutritional and Lifestyle Management

Dietary and lifestyle changes are proven methods to assist in management of diabetes and improving glycemic control.[5] Once a patient's eGFR falls below 60 mL/min/1.73 m², dietary assessment becomes even more important and it is recommended patients consult with a nutritionist to optimize diet.[5] This is not only for improvement in management of hyperglycemia, but also to ensure the patient's protein, potassium, and phosphorus intake is appropriate in the presence of CKD to prevent further advancement of disease.[5,9] Patients should be strictly limiting their dietary protein intake to daily recommended allowance of 0.8 g/kg per day.[4] Patients who maintain this target have slower progression of their CKD compared with those who exceed this recommended intake. Furthermore, nutritional assessment and counseling may also be useful in those who are overweight or obese being that most patients will require dramatic lifestyle changes to obtain optimal control over their disease. In those with diabetes and kidney disease, target body mass index should be within the normal range (18.5–24.9 kg/m^2).[8] Patients will ultimately need to implement a multifaceted approach to their care, including not only dietary changes, but also implementing an exercise regimen, smoking cessation, and self-monitoring of BP and blood glucose.[5,8]

Control of Hyperglycemia

To help prevent diabetic patients from developing microvascular complications, with specific regard to DKD, the mainstay of treatment is to maintain tight glucose control. Better glycemic control not only helps to slow the progression of diabetes, but also helps to prevent and slow the progression of its complications.[5] Lowering A1c levels as a means of improving glycemic control, and therefore improving outcomes, has been highly supported by multiple clinical trials, including the 3 landmark clinical trials that are often cited in support of this measure: Action to Control Cardiovascular Risk in Diabetes (ACCORD), Action in Diabetes and Vascular Disease (ADVANCE), and Veterans Affairs Diabetes Trial (VADT).[5] It is important to note that these trials were focused on cardiovascular outcomes as opposed to kidney-specific outcomes. The monitoring of hemoglobin A1c is something that can be easily used by nearly any provider to monitor and counsel a patient regarding their glycemic targets. Some providers also use glucose monitoring to direct diabetes management; therefore, both targets for hemoglobin A1c and blood glucose measurements are summarized in **Table 4**. Interestingly, intensive glycemic control, defined as hemoglobin A1c targets of less than 6.5%, has not shown a benefit with regard to kidney-related outcomes, but does increase risks of severe hypoglycemia, leading the National Kidney Foundation to recommend a target hemoglobin A1c of 7.0%.[9]

There are few studies that have examined the degree of recommended glycemic control in patients with ESRD; however, it does appear that the standard targets may not need to be as strict in those with ESRD compared with earlier stages of CKD, especially when patients have other comorbidities.[10] Generally speaking, the risks of hypoglycemia increase in later stages of CKD and ESRD in patients treated with insulin and other antihyperglycemic agents, which can increase morbidity.

The Role of Glucose-Lowering Medications

Although diet and exercise may initially be effective for patients to maintain glycemic control, as diabetes progresses medications will be indicated for continued

Table 4 Glycemic targets for management of diabetes mellitus	
Glycemic Targets	
Hemoglobin A1c	<7% per the American Diabetes Association 7% per the National Kidney Foundation
Preprandial (fasting) glucose	80–130 mg/dL
Peak postprandial glucose	<180 mg/dL

Data from Marathe PH, Gao HX, Close KL. American Diabetes Association standards of medical care in diabetes 2017. J Diabetes 2017;9(4):320–4; and National Kidney Foundation. KDOQI clinical practice guideline for diabetes and CKD: 2012 update. Am J Kidney Dis 2012;60(5):850–86.

management. Therapeutic options available to diabetic patients continue to expand, particularly with regard to oral agents. Although the goal when introducing antihyperglycemic agents is primarily to control glycemia, there are some antihyperglycemic agents that have direct benefits to the kidneys as well, which is discussed in more detail in the next section. It is important to keep in mind that medication management may become more challenging as DKD progresses because the presence of kidney disease often limits the number of agents that can be used, and many medications may need dosing adjustment. Additionally, glycemic targets also may need to be adjusted in those with advanced kidney disease, as hypoglycemia can have increasingly adverse effects on morbidity and mortality in these patients.[5]

Blood Pressure and Lipid Management

The emphasis on the use of lipid-lowering agents and antihypertensives in diabetic patients has been predominantly to reduce the risks of major cardiovascular complications. This is because, independently of each other, both diabetes and CKD increase risks for cardiovascular disease, and when found in combination the risks are even greater.[8]

Hypertension is one of the more common comorbidities in those with diabetes and is known to increase the rate of progression of kidney disease.[8] Therefore, treatment is recommended with strict targets. The standard target recommended by the National Kidney Foundation is maintaining a BP lower than 130/80 in patients with DKD; however, there is some controversy regarding this goal.[8] In those with diabetes, traditionally ACE inhibitors and ARBs are considered first-line management for hypertension due to their kidney protective properties.

In patients with diabetes and concomitant CKD or DKD, the use of lipid-lowering medications has shown significant benefits with regard to reducing and potentially preventing cardiovascular outcomes, such as stroke and myocardial infarction.[11] However, with regard to preventing progression of CKD-related outcomes, there has not been strong evidence to support that these agents play a significant role. Despite this, the use of lipid-lowering medications in those with diabetes and DKD continues to be recommended to prevent cardiovascular morbidity.[9]

PHARMACOLOGIC MANAGEMENT

There are a myriad of antihyperglycemic agents available now enabling care to be tailored to each patient individually. For the purpose of this discussion, we focus on those agents most commonly used and those with known renal benefits or specific renal-related concerns. Other agents available for use in patients with DKD have been excluded because of either lack of widespread use or lack of direct benefits with regard to renal outcomes.

Management of Hyperglycemia

Metformin is considered first-line treatment in diabetes in those for whom it is not contraindicated. Until recently, the recommendations for withholding metformin in those with CKD had been quite strict and were decided based on creatinine levels. However, in 2016, these recommendations were modified to focus on monitoring of eGFR as follows:

- Metformin is contraindicated in those with an eGFR less than 30 mL/min/1.73 m^2.
- Metformin should not be initiated in those with eGFR less than 45 mL/min/1.73 m^2.[5]

The American College of Radiology also recently modified their recommendations in 2015 supporting continued use of metformin in patients receiving iodinated contrast media as long as they did not meet another contraindication criteria for metformin use and had no signs or symptoms of acute kidney injury.[12] Additionally, metformin does not increase risk of hypoglycemia, which often makes it a safer choice for those in whom hypoglycemia is a concern.[10]

Among sulfonylureas, glipizide and glimepiride still may be used with caution in patients with DKD, as they do carry some risk of hypoglycemia; although, they are generally considered safe due to their short acting nature and hepatic metabolism that protects the kidney.[10,13] Glyburide is a long-acting sulfonylurea and puts patients at more significant risk for severe and prolonged hypoglycemia and, therefore, it is recommended to avoid use of glyburide in patients with DKD.[10] Meglitinides (nateglinide and repaglinide) have similar pharmacologic action to sulfonylureas, but they have a much shorter duration of action and are dosed with meals leading to less risk for hypoglycemia.[10] Because of this, these agents are becoming more commonly used, even in those with DKD. Of note, dose adjustment is required for nateglinide as DKD progresses.[14]

Pioglitazone does not technically require dosing adjustment in CKD and it does not cause hypoglycemia. However, it does carry the risk of causing fluid retention, which should be taken into account when treating those with more advanced DKD or ESRD due to the risk of heart failure and cardiac complications, especially those with hypoalbuminemia or nephrotic syndrome.[10,13,14]

Dipeptidyl peptidase-4 (DPP4) inhibitors and glucagonlike peptide-1 (GLP1) agonists function by similar mechanisms of action and have gained popularity among providers. DPP4 inhibitors and GLP1 receptor agonists have both been shown to have direct benefits on the kidney independent from improved glycemic control.[5] Of particular interest, the DPP4 inhibitor linagliptin has been shown to decrease albuminuria when given in combination with a RAAS inhibitor compared with RAAS inhibitor alone, and it was also shown to improve microvascular function.[15,16] More investigations are under way to continue to evaluate for evidence of renal protection with DPP4 inhibitor use. Of note, DPP4 inhibitors should be dose reduced according to their labels as DKD progresses and GLP1 agonists should be discontinued once kidney disease reaches stage 4.[13]

Sodium-glucose transporter 2 (SGLT2) inhibitors are the newest class of antidiabetic medications to enter the market. The effects they have on glycemic control may be reduced in those with DKD; however, they may still produce renal and cardiovascular benefits. In particular, they have been found to reduce intraglomerular pressure, renal tubular glucose reabsorption, and albuminuria.[5] In a study evaluating empagliflozin specifically, not only is the risk for cardiovascular events decreased, but data showed that its use was also associated with slowed progression of DKD to ESRD.[17] Likewise, a later trial with canagliflozin found similar results that decline in eGFR was slowed and urinary albumin excretion was decreased when compared with glimepiride.[18] These studies therefore support the use of SGLT2 inhibitors in those with DKD for both renal and cardiac benefits.

Despite the progress that has been made in development of safe and useful oral medications in DKD, insulin remains the preferred method of management in those with severe hyperglycemia and with advanced kidney disease.[10,13] Of note, it is critical to keep in mind that insulin doses may need to be reduced to prevent increasing risks of hypoglycemia in the context of progressing kidney disease. This is because, although insulin resistance increases in DKD, the rate of insulin metabolism decreases, thereby leading to prolonged duration of action of insulin in these patients.[10]

As kidney disease progresses, insulin may become the only viable option for patients, depending on other comorbidities and the decreasing utility of oral agents in advanced stages of kidney disease.

Management of Blood Pressure and Lipids

Microvascular complications of diabetes are often associated with other comorbidities; specifically, those with DKD are at increased risk for the development of cardiovascular disease (CVD).[5] Because of the impact hypertension has on progression of DKD, it is recommended that all diabetic patients with hypertension and DKD be prescribed an ACE inhibitor or ARB to maintain appropriate BP targets and reduce risk of progression to ESRD.[5] These agents have been found to have renal protective properties predominantly mediated via blood pressure–lowering effects. In a trial using irbesartan, an ARB, decrease in systolic BP to levels below 120 mm Hg was associated with decreased rate of progression of DKD to ESRD.[13] In fact, both ACE inhibitors and ARBs have been studied in multiple randomized controlled trials in diabetic patients with hypertension and both classes of antihypertensives have shown slowed progression of albuminuria, slowed loss of eGFR, and, therefore, slowed progression to ESRD, making them first-line antihypertensives in those with diabetes.[13] Interestingly, ACE inhibitors and ARBs are not recommended for primary prevention of DKD in normotensive patients who do not have albuminuria due to lack of data to support a benefit in this scenario.[9] Once the patient does start to show evidence of progression toward DKD, characterized by the development of albuminuria, it is then recommended to initiate an ACE inhibitor or ARB at that time, even if they remain normotensive, to both slow progression of DKD and mitigate risks of cardiovascular disease.[9]

As mentioned previously, the utility of lipid management in DKD at this time is directed primarily at preventing cardiovascular complications. Multiple clinical trials have shown significant cardiovascular benefits from the use of statins for control of hyperlipidemia in those with diabetes and DKD.[13] Additionally, a combination of statin plus ezetimibe has also demonstrated efficacy in reducing cardiovascular outcomes in patients with CKD with or without diabetes.[13] However, to date no studies have shown specific renal benefits with use of lipid-lowering agents. Of importance, in patients with ESRD, the cardiovascular benefits were found to be statistically nonsignificant and it is not recommended to initiate lipid-lowering medication, namely statins, in those who have already progressed to ESRD and are on dialysis due to the potential for serious adverse effects.[9,11]

LIMITATIONS, CONTROVERSIES, AND THE FUTURE OF MONITORING AND MANAGEMENT OF DIABETIC KIDNEY DISEASE

As with management of any medical condition, there are limitations to optimal management of kidney disease in patients with diabetes, from diagnosis and monitoring to pharmaceutical intervention.

Limitations in Monitoring

The major limitations to assessment are intrinsic limitations in measurements of the biomarkers commonly used for assessment of diabetes and DKD.

- eGFR is an estimated calculation and at best has a 90% chance of being within 30% of the true GFR
- As GFR increases, the calculation becomes less reliable, which can lead to early stages of DKD being missed

- Measurement of albuminuria is not standardized[4]
- A1c readings may be falsely lower in those with DKD and ESRD
- A1c readings also may be unreliable in other clinical conditions, such as anemia and hemolysis[10]

Furthermore, our current guidelines for predicting physiology of the development of DKD are not always consistent for each patient.

- Not all patients with DKD develop albuminuria with decreases in eGFR
- The degree of albuminuria can be affected by episodic hyperglycemia, alterations in BP, fever, urinary tract infection, and congestive heart failure, among others[4]

Controversies in Management

Additional limitations come in the form of management controversies. Of notable importance are differences in recommendations regarding BP targets, and when and how to use ACE inhibitors and ARBs properly.

Over the years, there have been multiple studies evaluating management of hypertension, including the National Kidney Foundation Kidney Disease Outcomes Quality Initiative and the findings from the ACCORD study group, from which the American Diabetes Association draws its recommendation.[9,19] These 2 sources have recommended differing BP goals: the former recommends maintaining BP lower than 130/80 mm Hg, whereas the latter recommends maintaining BP lower than 140/80 mm Hg.[20] The driving force for these differences was mostly related to study targets and characteristics of the study population. Although both looked at cardiovascular endpoints, ACCORD did not look at DKD-related targets, nor did their study population contain a sufficient number of participants with DKD. The ACCORD trial showed no benefit with regard to cardiovascular outcomes with intensive BP control, hence the recommendation for more modest targets.[19] However, there have been other smaller studies that have shown kidney benefits, namely slowed progression of DKD, with intensive BP control, characterized as BP <130 to 80 mm Hg.[20] Because it is unclear where the line is between increased benefit versus increased risk, there is currently a strong focus on tailoring goals to be specific to each patient depending on their other comorbidities. Therefore, it is generally recommended that if patients do not show signs of DKD, a target of 140/80 mm Hg should be sufficient, and in those cases with DKD more intensive targets should be aimed for, if they can be tolerated by the patient.[20]

ACE inhibitors and ARBs have been a mainstay of treatment for hypertensive patients with diabetes due to the significant effects they have repeatedly shown in slowing DKD progression. However, they are associated with initial increase in creatinine and decrease in eGFR, which may scare providers into discontinuing the medication early.[20] Studies have shown that initial increases in creatinine and decrease in eGFR may have positive prognostic indications for overall slowing of DKD progression in the long term.[20] Therefore, in those cases in which there is a modest initial drop in eGFR, these medications may not need to be discontinued immediately. Additional controversy surrounding the use of these medications is whether ACE inhibitors or ARBs are indicated for primary prevention of DKD. As mentioned before, currently there is not sufficient data to recommend use of these agents in normotensive patients with diabetes without evidence of DKD despite the existence of some evidence to suggest primary prevention may be effective.[20] Finally, the third controversy surrounding these agents is whether they should be used in combination with each other. There have been some studies that have shown improvement in kidney outcomes when patients are placed on combination therapy with an ACE inhibitor and an ARB. Unfortunately,

Table 5
Controversies and challenges in management of DKD

Topic	Controversy	Current Recommendation
Blood pressure targets	Major studies have recommended either a target of 140/80 mm Hg vs 130/80 mm Hg; which is preferred?	With regard to cardiovascular endpoints, no benefit is seen with intensive blood pressure control; however, if not contraindicated, intensive control may be preferred in patients with DKD.
When to initiate ACE inhibitors or ARBs	Is there utility of ACE inhibitors and ARBs for use in primary prevention of DKD?	ACE inhibitors and ARBs are not recommend for use in diabetic patients who are normotensive and have normal urine albumin excretion.
Use of ACE inhibitors and ARBs in combination	Should patients be recommended to take an ACE inhibitor and ARB together?	ACE inhibitors and ARBs should not be used in combination based on the current data.
When should ACE inhibitors and ARBs be discontinued	Increase in creatinine and decrease in eGFR is often seen on initiating these agents.	Long-term studies show initial increase in creatinine and decrease in eGFR may signify overall decrease in long-term progression of DKD. Further detailed studies about the use of these agents as CKD progresses is limited and they may be safe to continue even as patients transition to ESRD.
Use of calcium channel blockers	What is the role of calcium channel blockers in slowing progression of DKD (specifically compared with other antihypertensives)?	A calcium channel blocker should be used in addition to an ACE inhibitor or ARB when a second agent is indicated, as combination therapy shows decreased progression of albuminuria.
Role for lipid management	Does treating hyperlipidemia slow progression of DKD?	Studies have been positive regarding the use of fenofibrate in reducing albuminuria; more studies are needed to determine if treatment of hyperlipidemia prevents or slows DKD progression.
Diet and lifestyle	• Should low-protein diets be recommended? • What is the role of weight loss?	• High-protein diets are known to promote proteinuria; no benefit was seen in studies with restricted protein diets; therefore, the current recommendation is for maintaining the recommended daily intake of 0.8 g/kg/d. • There have been no studies to indicate that weight loss intrinsically slows progression of DKD or slowed DKD progression is seen due to the improvement in hyperglycemia and hypertension seen after weight loss.

Abbreviations: ACE, angiotensin-converting enzyme; ARB, angiotensin receptor blocker; CKD, chronic kidney disease; DKD, diabetic kidney disease; DM, diabetes mellitus; eGFR, estimated glomerular filtration rate; ESRD, end-stage renal disease.

Data from Stanton RC. Clinical challenges in diagnosis and management of diabetic kidney disease. Am J Kidney Dis 2014;63(2, Supplement 2):S3–21.

the VA NEPHRON-D study, which was evaluating the use of combination therapy, was halted prematurely because of increased incidences of acute kidney injury and hyperkalemia, calling into question safety risks of using both agents concomitantly.[20] The VALID study (Preventing ESRD in Overt Nephropathy of Type 2 Diabetes) also looked at the utility of combination therapy, although results have yet to be published.[20] Additional controversies are presented in **Table 5**.

The Future of Monitoring and Management of Diabetic Kidney Disease

As mentioned earlier in the article, the pathophysiology of DKD is complex and yet to be fully understood. At this time, the only available biomarkers for monitoring DKD are albuminuria and eGFR. Other biomarkers, such as serum uric acid and tumor necrosis factor receptor levels, have shown some promise in further assisting with the overall assessment and monitoring of DKD, but are not currently recommended for clinical use.[6] Further still, there are additional potential biomarkers of DKD progression that could be studied as well, including markers of oxidative stress, profibrotic cytokines, and advanced glycation end-products, that could prove useful in the future for monitoring and for determining prognosis.[6] Not only do we currently lack other biomarkers

Table 6
Areas of study for potential therapies for improved management of DKD

Pathophysiologic Target	Therapy Studied	Outcome
Vascular flow and anti-inflammatory effects	Pentoxifylline	Studies to date have been too small to make formal recommendations, although it does appear to decrease proteinuria.
RAAS pathway	Aldosterone inhibition: spironolactone	Multiple studies show decreased proteinuria with use of spironolactone; long-term studies will be needed to make formal conclusions.
RAAS pathway	Renin inhibition: aliskiren	Results are unclear to date.
Oxidative stress	Antioxidants vs placebo	Data suggestive of reduced progression to ESRD with antioxidant therapy.
Kinase pathways	"RBX": a PKC-β inhibitor (*Protein Kinase C*)	Improvement in albuminuria, GFR, and retinal circulation has been seen in rats, and a Phase II trial showed decreased albumin-to-creatinine ratio.
Advanced glycosylation end-products (AGEs)	Pyridoxamine (a vitamin B derivative)	Preserved kidney function seen in rats, and a Phase II trial in patients with DKD appears to reduce the rate of increase in creatinine and found reduced plasma AGE levels.
Anti-TNFα	Infliximab	Reduced urinary albumin excretion and delayed fibrosis has been seen in rats.

Abbreviations: DKD, diabetic kidney disease; ESRD, end-stage renal disease; GFR, glomerular filtration rate; RAAS, renin-angiotensin-aldosterone.
Data from Stanton RC. Clinical challenges in diagnosis and management of diabetic kidney disease. Am J Kidney Dis 2014;63(2, Supplement 2):S3–21; and Alicic RZ, Tuttle KR. Novel therapies for diabetic kidney disease. Adv Chronic Kidney Dis 2014;21(2):121–33.

that may assist with predicting risk of progression of DKD, but we are limited by the lack of pharmacologic agents that specifically target prevention of DKD progression. There are several mechanisms that could serve as targets for possible pharmaceutical development for better management in the future. A few potential therapies have already been studied, some with and some without success.[21] Of interest, the use of mineralocorticoid receptor antagonists for management of hypertension is becoming an area for further study due to recent evidence that they may reduce albuminuria, and therefore slow DKD progression.[5] However, there have been no long-term studies yet to support a formal recommendation for their use in DKD. Additional examples of potential pharmaceutical targets are outlined in **Table 6**.

SUMMARY

DKD is a complex microvascular complication of diabetes that poses challenging questions to providers about monitoring and management. In patients with diabetes, providers need to be diligent about close monitoring of albuminuria and eGFR for evidence of developing DKD so that interventions can begin as early as possible to reduce risks of not only further progression of DKD, but also to prevent cardiovascular complications. Management of DKD, much like diabetes itself, requires a multifaceted approach, including a combination of lifestyle modifications and pharmacologic intervention. Fortunately, many available oral antihyperglycemic agents are safe to use in DKD, and a few have even shown independent kidney protective benefits, namely SGLT2 inhibitors, DPP4 inhibitors, and GLP1 agonists. Likewise, the first-line agents recommended for hypertension in diabetes, ACE inhibitors and ARBs, also have independent kidney benefits. Despite all that has been accomplished in the management of DKD, there is still room for improvement and further studies are under way to discover new biomarkers that may further assist in diagnosis and prognosis of DKD, and new pharmacologic agents that directly target prevention and slowing progression of DKD.

REFERENCES

1. Boyle JP, Thompson TJ, Gregg EW, et al. Projection of the year 2050 burden of diabetes in the US adult population: dynamic modeling of incidence, mortality, and prediabetes prevalence. Popul Health Metr 2010;8(1):1.
2. Centers for Disease Control and Prevention. National diabetes statistics report: estimates of diabetes and its burden in the United States, 2014. Atlanta (GA): US Department of Health and Human Services; 2014. p. 1–12.
3. Centers for Disease Control and Prevention. National diabetes fact sheet: national estimates and general information on diabetes and prediabetes in the United States, 2011. Atlanta (GA): US Department of Health and Human Services, Centers for Disease Control and Prevention; 2011. p. 1–12.
4. Tuttle KR, Bakris GL, Bilous RW, et al. Diabetic kidney disease: a report from an ADA consensus conference. Am J Kidney Dis 2014;64(4):510–33.
5. Marathe PH, Gao HX, Close KL. American Diabetes Association standards of medical care in diabetes 2017. J Diabetes 2017;9(4):320–4.
6. MacIsaac RJ, Ekinci EI, Jerums G. Markers of and risk factors for the development and progression of diabetic kidney disease. Am J Kidney Dis 2014;63(2, Supplement 2):S39–62.
7. Arora MK, Singh UK. Molecular mechanisms in the pathogenesis of diabetic nephropathy: an update. Vascul Pharmacol 2013;58(4):259–71.

8. Saunders W. KDOQI clinical practice guidelines and clinical practice recommendations for diabetes and chronic kidney disease. 2007; 49(2, Supplement 2):S1-S180.

9. National Kidney Foundation. KDOQI clinical practice guideline for diabetes and CKD: 2012 update. Am J Kidney Dis 2012;60(5):850–86.

10. Williams ME, Garg R. Glycemic management in ESRD and earlier stages of CKD. Am J Kidney Dis 2014;63(2, Supplement 2):S22–38.

11. Slinin Y, Ishani A, Rector T, et al. Management of hyperglycemia, dyslipidemia, and albuminuria in patients with diabetes and CKD: a systematic review for a KDOQI clinical practice guideline. Am J Kidney Dis 2012;60(5):747–69.

12. Shah AD, McHargue C, Yee J, et al. Intravenous contrast in patients with diabetes on metformin: new common sense guidelines. Endocr Pract 2016;22(4):502–5.

13. Gosmanov AR, Wall BM, Gosmanova EO. Diagnosis and treatment of diabetic kidney disease. Am J Med Sci 2014;347(5):406–13.

14. Roche-Recinos A, Charlap E, Markell M. Management of glycemia in diabetic patients with stage IV and V chronic kidney disease. Curr Diab Rep 2015;15(5):25.

15. Jax T, Stirban A, Terjung A, et al. A randomised, active- and placebo-controlled, three-period crossover trial to investigate short-term effects of the dipeptidyl peptidase-4 inhibitor linagliptin on macro- and microvascular endothelial function in type 2 diabetes. Cardiovasc Diabetol 2017;16:13.

16. Groop P-H, Cooper ME, Perkovic V, et al. Linagliptin lowers albuminuria on top of recommended standard treatment in patients with type 2 diabetes and renal dysfunction. Diabetes Care 2013;36(11):3460–8.

17. Wanner C, Inzucchi SE, Lachin JM, et al. Empagliflozin and progression of kidney disease in type 2 diabetes. N Engl J Med 2016;375(4):323–34.

18. Heerspink HJ, Desai M, Jardine M, et al. Canagliflozin slows progression of renal function decline independently of glycemic effects. J Am Soc Nephrol 2017; 28(1):368–75.

19. ACCORD Study Group, Cushman WC, Evans GW, et al. Effects of intensive blood-pressure control in type 2 diabetes mellitus. N Engl J Med 2010;362: 1575–85.

20. Stanton RC. Clinical challenges in diagnosis and management of diabetic kidney disease. Am J Kidney Dis 2014;63(2, Supplement 2):S3–21.

21. Alicic RZ, Tuttle KR. Novel therapies for diabetic kidney disease. Adv Chronic Kidney Dis 2014;21(2):121–33.

Management of Diabetes in Children and Adolescents

Celia Levesque, RN, MSN, CNS-BC, NP-C, CDE, BC-ADM*

KEYWORDS

- Type 1 diabetes • Type 2 diabetes • Monogenic diabetes • Insulin and metformin
- Diabetes technology • Children • Adolescents

KEY POINTS

- Diabetes is among the most common chronic diseases in children and adolescents.
- Proper diagnosis of the type of diabetes in children and adolescents is important in order to implement an effective treatment plan.
- Technology to assist with diabetes treatment is advancing rapidly.
- A multidisciplinary pediatric diabetes team with the child/adolescent and caregiver at the center of the team is essential to achieve desired outcomes.

INTRODUCTION

Diabetes mellitus (DM) is the third most common disease in children and adolescents under 18 years of age (youth).[1] Managing DM in youth can be challenging because of factors such as physical growth, sexual maturity, family dynamics, developmental stages, and psychological adjustment as youth transition from being dependent to independent.[2] To achieve the best outcomes, it is necessary to have a multidisciplinary pediatric team of specialists including physicians/advanced practice providers, certified DM educators to teach diabetes self-management education (DSME) and medical nutrition therapy (MNT), and psychosocial support personnel with the patient and family[3,4] at the center of the team. Treatment plans will need to be revised frequently, so it is important that the team works together closely. This article will discuss the prevalence, diagnostic criteria, types, and treatment of DM in youth, as well as transitioning from pediatric to adult care.

PREVALENCE OF DIABETES IN YOUTH IN THE UNITED STATES

Most youth with DM have type 1 diabetes (T1DM); however, type 2 diabetes (T2DM) is becoming epidemic in youth. The prevalence of DM in youth in the United States was

Disclosure Statement: There are no commercial or financial conflicts of interest.
Department of Endocrine Neoplasia and Hormonal Disorders, MD Anderson Cancer Center, 1515 Holcomb Boulevard, Houston, TX 77030, USA
* 14726 Leighwood Creek Lane, Humble, TX 77396.
E-mail address: clevesqu@mdanderson.org

unknown until the early 2000s. The SEARCH for Diabetes in Youth study (SEARCH), an ongoing multicenter national study sponsored by the US Centers for Disease Control and Prevention (CDC) and The National Institute of Diabetes and Digestive and Kidney Diseases (NIDDK), was launched in 2000 and will continue until at least 2020 with the aim of discovering the prevalence of DM in youth in the United States.[5] The prevalence of T1DM in youth in 2001 was 1.48 cases per 1000 youth, and in 2009, it was 1.93 cases per 1000 youth, increasing by 21.1%. The prevalence of T2DM in youth in 2001 was 0.34 cases per 1000 youth in 2001, and in 2009 it was 0.46 cases per 1000 youth, increasing by 30.5%.[6]

DIAGNOSING DIABETES IN YOUTH

Diagnostic criteria for DM in youth are the same as for adults. The diagnosis is based on 1 of the following criteria:

- Hemoglobin A1c (HbA1c) of at least 6.5% performed by a National Glycohemoglobin Standardization Program (NGSP) laboratory standardized to the Diabetes Control and Complication Trial (DCCT) assay
- Fasting plasma glucose of at least 126 mg/dL (no caloric intake for at least 8 hours)
- Two-hour plasma glucose of at least 200 mg/dL during an oral glucose tolerance test using a glucose load containing 75 g anhydrous glucose dissolved in water
- Presence of classic symptoms of hyperglycemia or hyperglycemic crisis with a random plasma glucose of at least 200 mg/dL[3]

The laboratory results should be repeated if unequivocal hyperglycemia is absent. The American Diabetes Association (ADA) recommends using blood glucose rather than HbA1c to diagnose T1DM.[7]

TYPES OF DIABETES

Diabetes is classified into the following categories[3]:

- T1DM
- T2DM
- Gestational diabetes mellitus (GDM)
- Specific types of DM due to other causes

Gestational DM in youth will not be discussed in this article.

IMPORTANCE OF GLYCEMIC CONTROL

The current glycemic targets for DM are based on several key landmark trials. The Diabetes Control and Complications Trial (DCCT) was a randomized controlled trial conducted from 1982 to 1993 with 1441 subjects aged 13 to 39 years with T1DM, comparing conventional diabetes treatment (CON) with intensive insulin management (INT). Patients with hypertension, hypercholesterolemia, severe diabetic complications, or medical conditions were excluded. The subjects were also divided into a primary prevention arm for those with T1DM 1 to 5 years duration and without any diabetic retinopathy (DR) or urinary albumin excretion of at least 40 mg per 24 hours, and a secondary intervention arm for those with T1DM 1 to 15 years duration with mild-to-moderate DR. The patients in the CON arm of the study were treated with 1 to 2 daily insulin injections with daily urine or finger stick blood glucose monitoring (FSBG). No changes were made in their DM treatment plan unless the HbA1c exceeded 13.5%. The patients in the INT arm used at least 3 insulin injections per day or a continuous subcutaneous insulin infusion (CSII) pump with 4 or more FSBG tests per day. The patients were given a premeal target BG of 70 to 120 mg/dL and a 2-hour postprandial (PP) target of less than 180 mg/dL. Once weekly, a 3 AM FSBG was checked with a goal of greater than 65 mg/dL. Patients in the INT arm had frequent interaction with the clinical staff for treatment adjustments and education. The results of the study showed that The INT arm achieved a mean HbA1c of 7.2% compared with 9.1% with the CON arm. The DM complications that were monitored during the study included DR, albuminuria, and diabetic neuropathy. The results showed a reduction of the development of several complications in the INT arm compared with the CON arm:

- DR reduced by 76% in the primary prevention group and 54% in the secondary intervention group
- Microalbuminuria (urine albumin excretion ≥40 mg per 24 hours) reduced by 39% in the primary and secondary groups combined
- Albuminuria (urine albumin excretion ≥300 mg per 24 hours) reduced by 54% in the primary and secondary groups combined
- Clinical neuropathy by 60% in the primary and secondary groups combined

The adverse event in the INT arm was a two- to threefold increase in severe hypoglycemia events compared with the CON arm.[8]

After the DCCT was completed, participants in the CON arm of the study were encouraged to switch to INT with the goal of improving their glycemic control. The CON group had a reduction of HbA1c from 9.1% to 8.1%, and the INT arm, no longer followed intensively by the researchers, had an increase of the HbA1c from 7.2% to 7.9%, resulting in a narrowing of the HbA1c gap between the 2 arms. The DCCT trial participants were followed after the study ended. The Epidemiology of Diabetes Interventions and Complications (EDIC) trial was conducted from 1994 to 2006 and studied 94% of the DCCT trial participants with a mean follow-up of 16 years. During the EDIC trial, 96% of the participants were retained. The goal of EDIC was to examine the long-term effects of the DCCT interventions on cardiovascular disease, retinopathy, renal disease, and neuropathy. **Table 1** shows the risk reduction of the INT arm compared with the CON arm that continued after the DCCT concluded, which shows that tight glycemic control early in the disease process has a legacy effect, reducing the rate of DM complications years later, even if the glycemic control deteriorates.

The EDIC trial investigated cardiovascular outcomes of the DCCT participants 30 years after conclusion of the DCCT. Subjects in the INT arm and those with lower levels of HbA1c had thinner carotid intima-media thickness as measured by ultrasound, coronary artery calcification with computed tomography, and cardiac structure and function with cardiac MRI.[10] Overall, the DCCT and EDIC showed that chronic hyperglycemia and duration of DM are the major risk factors in the pathogenies of microvascular complications in T1DM, and plays a role in the development of atherosclerosis.

GLYCEMIC GOALS IN YOUTH

For most youth, several glycemic goals are recommended:

- HbA1c less than 7.5%
- Premeal blood glucose 90 to 130 mg/dL
- Bedtime/overnight blood glucose 90 to 150 mg/dL[7]

Individualized glycemic targets should be based on the risk of hypoglycemia. A higher target may be needed if frequent or severe hypoglycemia occurs.[7] Individuals

Table 1
Risk reduction with intensive insulin management compared with conventional diabetes treatment in the epidemiology of diabetes interventions and complications trial

Complication	Percent Risk Reduction During DCCT	Percent Risk Reduction During EDIC
DR 3-step change	63	72
DR proliferative	47	76
Macular edema	26	77
Laser treatment	51	77
Microalbuminuria (>28 mg/min)	39	53
Albuminuria (>208 mg/min)	54	82
Neuropathy	60	Assessment of neuropathy different in EDIC compared with DCCT precluding comparison[9]

with a lower C-peptide have a higher risk for hypoglycemia than those with higher C-peptides. Children younger than 6 years may not be able to recognize and/or tell a caregiver about symptoms of hypoglycemia. Hypoglycemia may cause subtle neurocognitive impairment in children including deficits on perceptual, motor, memory, and attention tasks. Those younger than 5 years and those who have seizures are at a higher risk.[11]

TYPE 1 DIABETES IN YOUTH

T1DM is an immune-mediated loss of pancreatic beta (β) cells leading to absolute insulin deficiency in genetically susceptible people who have an environmental trigger. It is associated with HLA DQA and DQB genes. The time from the beginning of the β-cell attack to the development of hyperglycemia can vary greatly in individuals with T1DM but tends to be shorter in infants and young children. Within 5 to 10 years after diagnosis of T1DM, β-cell loss is complete, and circulating islet cell autoantibodies are undetectable.[12] Hyperglycemia develops when 80% to 90% of the β-cells have been destroyed, as illustrated in **Fig. 1**.

The risk for development of T1DM in those who have 3 to 4 positive autoantibodies is 60% to 100% in 5 to 10 years.[13] Persistence of 2 or more autoantibodies islet cell autoantibodies, glutamate decarboxylase 2 enzyme (GAD65), islet antigen-2 (IA-2) and islet antigen 2 beta (IA-2β) and zinc transporter 8 (ZnT8) predicts clinical T1DM.[7] Because T1DM is autoimmune, patients are more prone to the development of other autoimmune disorders. The symptoms of T1DM, including polyuria, polydipsia, polyphagia, and weight loss, are often severe. Many will have diabetic ketoacidosis (DKA) at diagnosis. In children younger than age 2, 40% will have DKA at diagnosis and approximately 5% of those will die.[12] Environmental triggers may play a role because of

- Less than 10% of individuals with HLA-conferred DM develop overt T1DM
- There is less than a 40% concordance rate among monozygotic twins
- There is a tenfold difference in the incidence among Caucasians in Europe
- There has been a dramatic increase in incidence over the past 50 years
- The incidence increases in population groups that have moved from an area of low incidence to high incidence.[13]

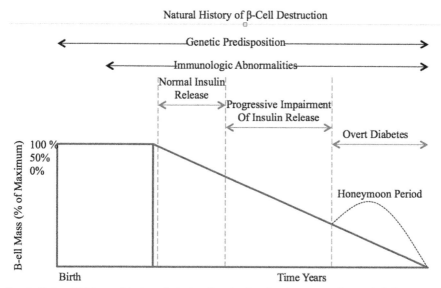

Fig. 1. Natural history of beta-cell destruction in the development of type 1 diabetes.

Some of the suspected triggers include viruses such as coxsackie B4, enterovirus, togavirus, rubella, mumps, rotavirus, parvovirus, and cytomegalovirus,[14] cow's milk-based formula ingestion as an infant, and environmental toxins.[12] There are 3 stages to the development of T1DM:

1. Positive multiple autoantibodies with normoglycemia and no symptoms
2. All characteristics of stage 1 plus BG levels in the prediabetes criteria with no symptoms
3. Overt DM meeting diagnostic criteria with clinical symptoms[7]

Initiation of insulin therapy in patients with T1DM may cause a transient remission or partial remission in T1DM referred to as a honeymoon.[3,12,15] Existing β-cells at diagnosis temporally increase insulin secretion causing a decreased need for exogenous insulin. The honeymoon phase does not occur in all newly diagnosed youth, and the duration is variable. Most will still require insulin therapy to maintain normoglycemia. A prospective study of 103 children younger than 12 years of age reported the frequency, duration, and factors that affect remission (honeymoon). Of the 103 patients, 71 experienced partial remission; 3 of the 71 patients experienced complete remission. The average time to remission was 28.6 days plus or minus 12.3 days. Children older than 5 and those with lower BG levels at diagnosis had a higher rate of remission, and children with DKA or long duration of symptoms prior to diagnosis had lower rates of remission.[15]

Treatment of Type 1 Diabetes Mellitus

The basic components of treating T1DM in youth include

- Care provided by a multidisciplinary pediatric team specializing in the care of T1DM in youth
- Diabetes self-management education for the patient and caregivers that is appropriate for the child's developmental needs and culturally sensitive

- Medical nutritional therapy focusing on carbohydrate counting
- Physiologic insulin replacement utilizing a basal-prandial-correctional regimen
- Ongoing assessment of family stressors, psychosocial distress, and mental health problems including fear of hypoglycemia, depression, anxiety, and disordered eating
- Assess for other autoimmune disease associated with T1DM
  - Assess for thyroid disease: test antithyroid peroxidase and antithyroglobulin antibodies soon after diagnosis, and test TSH soon after diagnosis, after glucose control has been achieved, if there are symptoms of thyroid dysfunction, and every 1 to 2 years if there are no symptoms
  - Assess for celiac disease; consider measuring tissue transglutaminase or deamidated gliadin antibodies, with documentation of normal total serum immunoglobulin A (IgA) levels soon after diagnosis, and in patients with or their first-degree relatives with
    - Celiac disease
    - Growth failure
    - Weight loss
    - Failure to gain weight
    - Diarrhea
    - Flatulence
    - Abdominal pain
    - Signs of malabsorption
    - Frequent unexplained hypoglycemia or worsening glucose control[7]

Depending on the age of the youth, various developmental issues affect the treatment plan (**Table 2**).

Physiologic Insulin Replacement in the Treatment of Type 1 Diabetes

In individuals without DM, glucose is the main stimulator of insulin release from the pancreatic β-cell. First-phase insulin, in response to nutrient and non-nutrient secretagogues, is a burst of insulin lasting only a few minutes. Second-phase insulin release is in response only to nutrients. Basal insulin is the small, continuous amount of insulin that suppresses hepatic glucose output during the fasting state. Most youth with T1DM are treated with an intensive insulin therapy regimen using multiple daily insulin injections or an insulin pump. The purpose of intensive insulin therapy is to mimic normal physiologic insulin secretion. The total daily insulin requirement for most individuals with T1DM is 0.4 to 1 unit per kilogram weight, with a typical starting dose of 0.5 units per kilogram, with approximately 50% as basal insulin and 50% as bolus insulin. Insulin doses are adjusted based on glucose patterns. Youth who are extremely active may require less basal insulin and more bolus insulin compared with less active youth. Rapid- or short-acting insulin is used for treatment of food. Most use insulin-to-carbohydrate ratio to calculate the meal dose. Rapid- or short-acting insulin is used to correct hyperglycemia.[17] The onset, peak, and duration of insulins are presented in **Table 3**.

Technology in the Treatment of Diabetes in Youth

Glucose meters

Glucose meters are small, portable, accurate, and fast; they require small sample sizes, and some have the ability to communicate via Bluetooth technology to phone applications.

Table 2
Developmental issues in the treatment of type 1 diabetes in youth

Age years	Issues
Infants 0–1	Requires frequent feeding, monitoring, and injections. It is difficult for caregivers to differentiate irritability from hypoglycemia from the usual causes.
Toddlers 1–3	Unpredictable eating patterns. They are starting to feed themselves, so let them choose from generally healthy foods. Let the child choose the finger for finger sticks, injection site, and let them help as they are capable.
Preschool 3–5	This age may view DM treatment as a punishment and may be very fearful. Teach child to report symptoms of hypoglycemia and what to eat when low. Teach all caregivers how to recognize and treat hypoglycemia. Allow child to perform simple tasks such as putting a drop of blood on the strip if he or she wishes.
School 5–12	Teach all school personnel about the DM treatment plan. Parents need to learn insulin adjustment. Encourage the child to participate in supervised self-care as he or she is capable. Shared family responsibility. Will need frequent insulin dose changes during periods of growth.
Adolescents	Diabetes management becomes more difficult as the adolescent becomes more independent, and peer relationships become more important. Diabetes treatment, when around others outside their family, may be omitted so as to not draw attention to the DM. BG control becomes more difficult during puberty because of hormone changes. Need to have family support and supervision as the adolescent slowly gains independence. Prepare the adolescent for gradually gaining independence and transitioning to adulthood.

Data from Refs.[2,3,12,16]

Betahydroxybuterate meters

Betahydroxybuterate (β-OHB) meters are available to check for blood ketones. Testing blood ketones during illness or with extreme hyperglycemia is a more accurate way to detect DKA early. When individuals develop DKA, the ketone body accumulation is acetoacetate (AcAc) and β-OHB, which has an acid property. The β-OHB is generated by the reduction of AcAc in mitochondria, and acetone develops by decarboxylation of AcAc. Acetone does not possess acidic property. With DKA, the ratio of serum β-OHB to AcAc is usually 1:1 to 10:1. Urine ketone testing products use a nitroprusside reaction, which tests for acetone and does not detect β-OHB; therefore the early diagnosis of DKA may be missed.[18] The disadvantage to using a β-OHB meter is that the test is expensive, costing approximately $5 per strip. Two meters on the market are able to test for β-OHB: the Precision X-tra, and the NovoMax; both are equally easy to use and require less than 1 minute for results.

Continuous glucose sensors

A continuous glucose sensor is a catheter placed under the skin, usually in the abdominal area, that measures interstitial fluid glucose continuously and transmits the data to a receiver. Depending on the brand, the receiver may be a stand-alone receiver, a smart phone, or an insulin pump. Currently 2 companies produce continuous glucose monitors on the US market. Dexcom produces a G4 transmitter that communicates to a G4 receiver, the Animas insulin pump, or the Tandem insulin pump. The G4 receiver can transmit to a compatible cell phone. They also produce a G5 transmitter that can communicate to a compatible smart phone without a receiver or to a G5 receiver if the

Table 3
Peak, onset, and duration of insulins on the US market

Generic Name	Brand Name	Onset	Peak	Duration
Rapid Acting Insulin				
Aspart U-100	Novolog	5–15 min	45–75 min	2–4 h
Glulisine U-100	Apidra	5–15 min	45–75 min	2–4 h
Lispro U-100	Humalog	5–15 min	45–75 min	2–4 h
Lispro U-200	Humalog	5–15 min	45–75 min	2–4 h
Short-Acting Insulin				
Regular U-100	Humulin R Novolin R Relion R	60 min	2–4 h	5–8 h
Regular U-500	Humulin U-500	30 min	8 h	12–24 h
Intermediate-Acting Insulin				
NPH U-100	Humulin N Novolin N Relion N	2 h	4–12 h	18–28 h
NPL U-100	Found as part of premixed insulin	2 h	6 h	15 h
Basal Insulin				
Degludec U-100	Tresiba U-100		Peakless	Over 42 h
Degludec U-200	Tresiba U-200		Peakless	Over 42 h
Detemir U-100	Levemir	2 h	3–9 h	6–24 h
Glargine U-100	Lantus	2 h	Peakless	24 h
Glargine U-300	Toujeo	2 h	Peakless	24 + hrs

user does not have a compatible cell phone. Both the G4 and G5 sensors are US Food and Drug Administration (FDA) approved for 7-day wearing; both can share data with a significant other's compatible cell phone, and both are indicated for children age 2 and older. Only the Dexcom G5 system is FDA approved to be used as a finger stick replacement for DM treatment decisions. The Enlite sensor is approved for age 16 and older and has the ability to communicate to a receiver or to the Medtronic brand insulin pump. It is FDA approved for 6-day wearing; however, it does not have an indication as a finger stick replacement. All of the continuous sensors on the market have the capability to be programmed to alarm if the blood glucose level is too high or low.

Insulin pens
Most of the insulin brands on the US market come in the form of both a vial and a pen (**Table 4**). Insulin pens are convenient, accurate, and easy to use. Some of the pens are disposable, while others hold cartridges that are replaced.

Insulin pumps
Insulin pumps continuously deliver rapid-acting insulin similar to how the pancreas secretes insulin. The basal rate is the automatic continuous amount of insulin delivered to maintain target BG ranges when the wearer is fasting. Multiple basal rates can be programmed to adjust for varying basal requirements. A bolus is delivered to manage BG when the wearer is eating and to correct hyperglycemia. Although an innovative technology, children require supportive caregivers to assist with supervising the use of the pump. Many of the insulin pumps on the US market have features including

Table 4
Insulin pens available on the US market

Brand Name	Units per Disposable Pen/Cartridge	Disposable or Replaceable Cartridges	Unit Dose Range	Unit Measurement Increment
Apidra Solostar	300 units per pen 5 pens per box	Disposable	1–80	1
Autopen Classic Model AN3810	300 units per cartridge 5 cartridges per box	Cartridges	1–21	1
Autopen Classic Model AN3800	300 units per cartridge 5 cartridges per box	Cartridges	2–42	2
Humalog KwikPen	300 units per pen 5 pens per box	Disposable	1–60	1
Humalog U-200 KwikPen	600 units per pen 2 pens per box	Disposable	1–60	1
Humalog 50/50 KwikPen	300 units per pen 5 pens/box	Disposable	1–60	1
Humalog 75/25 KwikPen	300 units per pen 5 pens per box	Disposable	1–60	1
HumaPen Luxura HD	300 units per cartridge 5 cartridges per box	Cartridges	0.5–30	0.5
Humulin N Pen	300 units per pen 5 pens per box	Disposable	1–60	1
Humulin 70/30 Pen	300 units per pen 5 pens per box	Disposable	1–60	1
Humulin R U-500 Kwikpen	1500 units per pen 2 pens per box; 5 pens per box	Disposable	5–300	5
Lantus Solostar	300 units per pen 5 pens per box	Disposable	1–80	1
Levemir FlexTouch	300 units per pen 5 pens per box	Disposable	1–80	1
Novolog FlexPen	300 units per pen 5 pens per box	Disposable	1–60	1
Novolog Mix 70/30	300 units per pen 5 pens per box	Disposable	1–60	1
NovoPen Echo	300 units per cartridge 5 cartridges per box	Cartridges	0.5–30	0.5
Ryzodeg 70/30	300 units per pen 5 pens per box	Disposable	1–80	1
Toujeo Solostar	450 units per pen 3 pens per box	Disposable	1–80	1
Tresiba	300 units per pen 5 pens per box	Disposable	1–80	1
Tresiba U-200	600 units per pen 3 pens per box	Disposable	1–160	2

- Delivering insulin in very small increments, which makes delivering insulin more accurate
- Delivering a bolus in a variable manner in order to match the meal composition and gastric emptying time

- Communicating with a continuous glucose monitor, displaying the result on the screen
- Downloading insulin pump information for analysis and adjustment

The individual should select the brand of insulin pump that best meets his or her needs. All of the insulin pumps with the exception of the MiniMed 670G require the patient/caregiver to make adjustments in the basal and bolus doses based on BG patterns.

Hydrid closed loop insulin pump

The MiniMed 670G hybrid closed loop insulin pump system was FDA approved September 28, 2016, and released to the US market in 2017. It is indicated for ages 14 and older, and is contraindicated for individuals younger than 7 years of age and in individuals requiring less than 8 units of insulin per day. The hybrid closed loop insulin pump differs from all other insulin pumps in that when used in the automatic mode, the CGM communicates with the insulin pump and adjusts the basal rate to achieve target glucose levels. The user must bolus the insulin pump 20 minutes prior to consuming carbohydrates. In a study of the safety and effectiveness of this insulin pump, 32 of the 52 participants were adolescents with T1DM. The adolescents were found to have improved mean plasma glucose with less frequent hypoglycemia episodes using the automated insulin pump compared with using a nonautomated insulin pump. Studies using the system with children are underway.[19]

TYPE 2 DIABETES IN YOUTH

The incidence of T2DM in youth in the United States has dramatically increased in the past 20 years, and the estimated incidence is approximately 5000 new cases per year. T2DM in youth is associated with increased adiposity, family history, female sex, low socioeconomic status, and ethnic and racial minorities. Diagnosing T2DM in youth may be challenging, because youth with T1DM may be obese, and those with T2DM may have ketones and DM-related autoantibodies at diagnosis. Approximately 6% have DKA at diagnosis. Screen for T2DM in youth age 10 years or greater or puberty (if it occurs before age 10), in overweight youth with a body mass index (BMI) greater than the 85th percentile for age and sex, weight for height greater than the 85th percentile, or weight greater than 120% of ideal for height plus 2 of the following risk factors

- Family history of T2DM in a first- or second-degree relative
- Race/ethnicity in high risk group: Native American, African American, Latino, Asian American, Pacific Islander
- Signs of insulin resistance: acanthosis nigricans, hyperlipidemia, hypertension, polycystic ovary syndrome, or small-for-gestational-age birth weight

If the screening is normal, repeat screening every 3 years.[7] Because most youth with type 2 diabetes are obese, they are prone to comorbidities that increase cardiovascular disease including hypertension, hyperlipidemia, nonalcoholic fatty liver disease, and metabolic syndrome.[20] Youth with T2DM have a more rapidly progressive decline in β-cell function and have a more rapid development of DM complications when compared to adults with T2DM.[7]

Treatment of Type 2 Diabetes in Youth

Although glycemic goals are the same, treatment of T2DM in youth is different than treatment of T1DM. The goal of treatment is to achieve glycemic targets and prevent or treat comorbid conditions common to T2DM in youth including obesity, sleep apnea, hyperlipidemia, hypertension, and hepatic steatosis. Treatment includes the following

- Nutrition counseling for weight management
- Moderate-to-vigorous exercise at least 60 minutes per day
- Limit nonacademic screen time to less than 2 hours per day
- Metformin is initiated at diagnosis if there are no contraindications, ketosis, DKA, questionable diagnosis of T1DM, BG of at least 250 or HbA1c greater than 9%. Initiate 500 mg by mouth daily and titrate the dose up by 500 mg every 1 to 2 weeks as tolerated. Extended-release metformin has a reduced incidence of gastrointestinal adverse effects compared with immediate-release
- Insulin is initiated in patients with ketosis or DKA, questionable diagnosis of T1DM, or a random BG of at least 250 mg/dL or HbA1c greater than 9%
- The HbA1c should be monitored every 3 months, and the patient should check FSBG if taking insulin, changing the DM regimen, or in those not meeting HbA1c targets

When initiating insulin therapy in a patient already taking metformin, begin with 1 daily injection of a basal insulin (see **Table 3**) and twice daily FSBG monitoring, preferably fasting and one 2-hour postprandial. If the patient does not achieve glycemic targets with metformin and basal insulin, then prandial insulin (see **Table 3**) should be added to the regimen. Insulin to carbohydrate ratio with a correctional scale can be implemented if the patient/family is willing to count grams of carbohydrate and perform FSBG testing prior to eating in order to determine the correct insulin dose. The use of an insulin pump can be an option if the patient and family desire to use the insulin pump and meet criteria. Unfortunately less than 10% of youth with T2DM will be able to achieve glycemic targets with therapeutic lifestyle modifications alone. Compliance to therapy and follow-up is reduced in patients not taking DM medications. The perception of DM is more serious if medications are used.[21] See **Table 5** to differentiate the characteristics between T1DM and T2DM.

MONOGENIC DIABETES SYNDROMES

Monogenic DM is characterized by defects in β-cell functioning, impairing insulin secretion with minimal or no defects in insulin action. Inheritance is by an autosomal-dominant pattern involving the following chromosomes

- 12 in the hepatic transcription factor hepatocyte nuclear factor-1β
- 7p in the glucokinase gene
- 20q in the hepatic transcription factor HNF-4β

It is usually diagnosed before the age of 25 and presents with mild hyperglycemia. Leprechaunism and Rabson-Mendenhall syndrome are pediatric syndromes that have mutations in the insulin receptor gene with alterations in insulin receptor function causing extreme insulin resistance. Both are extremely rare.[12] Monogenic DM accounts for 1% to 4% of pediatric cases of DM. Because T1DM is rare in patients younger than 6 months, all who are diagnosed with DM in the first 6 months of life and those with negative antibodies who are 6 to 12 months need to have molecular genetic testing for neonatal diabetes mellitus (NDM). Testing will guide treatment. For example, those with a potassium channel mutation can be treated with

Table 5
Characteristics of type 1 and type 2 diabetes mellitus

Characteristics	Type 1	Type 2
Previously named	Juvenile-onset, insulin-dependent diabetes, type 1 diabetes	Adult onset, noninsulin-dependent diabetes, type 2 diabetes
Screening	None in the mass population; consider in antibody testing in first-degree relatives	Consider in youth who are overweight or obese who have 2 or more additional diabetes risk factors
Race at highest risk	Caucasian	African American, Native American, Hispanic
Prevalence	1.93 per 1000 youth	0.46 per 1000 youth
Diagnostic test(s)	Blood glucose	Blood glucose or HbA1c
Pathophysiology	Progressive autoimmune attack of pancreatic β-cells leading to absolute insulin deficiency	Progressive insulin resistance with defective insulin secretion insufficient to compensate for the resistance
Beta-cell antibodies	Usually positive	Usually negative
Weight	Usually thin	Usually overweight
Signs/symptoms	Severe, sudden/polyuria, polydipsia, polyphagia, weight loss	Mild, slow progression/acanthosis nigricans
Ketones	Often positive at diagnosis	Often negative at diagnosis
Insulin production	Usually absent 5–10 y after diagnosis	Usually continues
Treatment	Must take insulin to survive	Metformin or insulin
Diabetic ketoacidosis	High risk for development if insulin omitted or during periods of increased stress	Lower risk compared with T1DM but can occur at diagnosis and during periods of increase stress
Risk for other autoimmune disorders	Hashimoto thyroiditis, Graves, Addison, and celiac disease, vitiligo, autoimmune hepatitis, myasthenia gravis, and pernicious anemia	No increased risk

high-dose sulfynolureas. Maturity onset diabetes of the young (MODY) is the most common form of monogenic DM and may be easily misdiagnosed as T1DM. Suspect MODY in patients with one of the following

- A first-degree relative with DM with no autoantibodies, low or no insulin requirements 5 years after diagnosis, and the lack of characteristics of T2DM such as obesity, acanthosis nigricans, and insulin resistance
- Mild stable fasting hyperglycemia with preserved β-cell functioning
- Absence of characteristics of T2DM in the patient
- Absence of islet autoantibodies[22]

Many subsets of monogenic DM exist that are associated with unique other clinical features. The diagnosis and treatment of monogenic DM require a specialist and will not be discussed in this article.

Transitioning

Although the diagnosis of DM is devastating, most youth and their families adjust well. Shifting from adolescence to adulthood requires adequate preparation. The ADA published a position statement for recommendations for transitioning from pediatric to adulthood DM care systems. They defined emerging adulthood as age 18 to 30 years. Many psychosocial adjustments occur during the emerging adulthood period. The individual may participate in risky behavior such as smoking, drinking alcohol, taking drugs, disordered eating, and having unprotected sex. As the emerging adult becomes independent, a busy lifestyle (eg, school, work, relationships) can take precedence over DM self-care. The patient often misses medical visits. Many will feel overwhelmed with the complexity of treatment and develop DM burnout. Worry, anxiety, and depression over poor DM control and the risk of developing acute and chronic DM complications are common and worsen glycemic control. Increased duration of DM increases the risk of DM complications.[2] The SEARCH trial showed that only 32% of youth age 13 to 18 years and 18% of those 19 years and older achieved a HbA1c of 7% or less.[1] The ADA recommendations for care transition for the emerging adult with DM includes

- A team approach with the pediatric DM team, patient, and family to prepare the emerging adult at least 1 year prior to the transfer to adult health
- The pediatric provider should refer the emerging adult to an adult provider and provide a written treatment plan for the emerging adult to take to the adult provider
- Inform the emerging adult about the differences in the care by a pediatric team versus an adult provider
- The focus of the transition should be on the emerging adult taking on more responsibilities for self-care skills including making their own DM appointments, making sure they have all of their DM medications and testing supplies, and carrying out the DM self-care activities needed to achieve glycemic targets
- Education on birth control, pregnancy planning, prevention of sexually transmitted diseases, use of alcohol and drugs, and driving precautions should be provided
- Those using insulin should have follow-up every 3 months, and patients with T2DM not on insulin should have visits every 3 to 6 months
- Screen for DM complications according to national guidelines
- Screen for psychosocial issues such as eating disorders and depression; refer to a mental health provider if needed

SUMMARY

Management of DM in youth is challenging. Although there is no cure for DM, emerging technology and pharmaceuticals make treatment easier. Youth require the support of caregivers. A team of diabetes specialists should provide education and support as the child transitions from with the patient/caregivers at the center of the team.

REFERENCES

1. Pettitt DJ, Talton J, Dabelea D, et al. Prevalence of diabetes in US youth in 2009: the SEARCH for diabetes in youth study. Diabetes Care 2014;37(2):402–8.

2. Peters A, Laffel L, American Diabetes Association Transitions Working Group. Diabetes care for emerging adults: recommendations for transition from pediatric to adult diabetes care systems. Diabetes Care 2011;34(11):2477–85.

3. Marathe PH, Gao HX, Close KL. American Diabetes Association standards of medical care in diabetes 2017. Diabetes Care 2017;40(S1):S1–135.

4. Powers MA, Bardsley J, Cypress M, et al. Diabetes self-management education and support in type 2 diabetes: a joint position statement of the American Diabetes Association, the American Association of Diabetes Educators, and the Academy of Nutrition and Dietetics. Diabetes Educ 2017;43(1):40–53.

5. Crume TL, Hamman RF, Isom S, et al. Factors influencing time to case registration for youth with type 1 and type 2 diabetes: SEARCH for Diabetes in Youth Study. Ann Epidemiol 2016;26(9):631–7.

6. Dabelea D, Mayer-Davis EJ, Saydah S, et al. Prevalence of type 1 and type 2 diabetes among children and adolescents from 2001 to 2009. JAMA 2014;311(17): 1778–86.

7. Marathe PH, Gao HX, Close KL. American Diabetes Association Standards of Medical Care in Diabetes 2017. J Diabetes 2017;9(4):320–4.

8. Diabetes Control and Complications Trial Research Group. The effect of intensive treatment of diabetes on the development and progression of long-term complications in insulin-dependent diabetes mellitus. N Engl J Med 1993;1993(329): 977–86.

9. Epidemiology of Diabetes Interventions and Complications (EDIC). Design, implementation, and preliminary results of a long-term follow-up of the Diabetes Control and Complications Trial cohort. Diabetes Care 1999;22(1):99–111.

10. Gao Y, Yoon KH, Chuang L-M, et al. Efficacy and safety of exenatide in patients of Asian descent with type 2 diabetes inadequately controlled with metformin or metformin and a sulphonylurea. Diabetes Res Clin Pract 2009;83(1):69–76.

11. Rovet JF, Ehrlich RM. The effect of hypoglycemic seizures on cognitive function in children with diabetes: a 7-year prospective study. J Pediatr 1999;134(4):503–6.

12. Kaufman FR. Medical management of type 1 diabetes. Alexandria (VA): American Diabetes Association; 2012.

13. Knip M, Veijola R, Virtanen SM, et al. Environmental triggers and determinants of Type 1 diabetes. Diabetes 2005;54(suppl 2):S125–36.

14. van der Werf N, Kroese FG, Rozing J, et al. Viral infections as potential triggers of type 1 diabetes. Diabetes Metab Res Rev 2007;23(3):169–83.

15. Abdul-Rasoul M, Habib H, Al-Khouly M. 'The honeymoon phase' in children with type 1 diabetes mellitus: frequency, duration, and influential factors. Pediatr Diabetes 2006;7(2):101–7.

16. Schreiner B. Diabetes education in hospitalized children: developmental and situational concerns. Crit Care Nurs Clin North Am 2013;25(1):101–9.

17. Association Diabetes Association. Practical insulin: a handbook for prescribing providers. Alexandria (VA): American Diabetes Association; 2015.

18. Lertwattanarak R, Plainkum P. Efficacy of quantitative capillary beta-hydroxybutyrate measurement in the diagnosis of diabetic ketoacidosis: a comparison to quantitative serum ketone measurement by nitroprusside reaction. J Med Assoc Thai 2014;97(Suppl 3):78–85.

19. Bergenstal RM, Garg S, Weinzimer SA, et al. Safety of a hybrid closed-loop insulin delivery system in patients with type 1 diabetes. JAMA 2016;316(13):1407–8.

20. Pinhas-Hamiel O, Zeitler P. Acute and chronic complications of type 2 diabetes mellitus in children and adolescents. Lancet 2007;369(9575):1823–31.

21. Copeland KC, Silverstein J, Moore KR, et al. Management of newly diagnosed type 2 diabetes mellitus (T2DM) in children and adolescents. Pediatrics 2013; 131(2):364–82.
22. Rubio-Cabezas O, Hattersley AT, Njølstad PR, et al. The diagnosis and management of monogenic diabetes in children and adolescents. Pediatr Diabetes 2014; 15(Suppl 20):47–64.

Management of Lipids in Patients with Diabetes

Ngozi D. Mbue, PhD, RN, ANP-C[a,b,c,]*, John E. Mbue, PharmD, MS, BCOP[b],
Jane A. Anderson, PhD, RN, FNP-C, FAAN[a,b,c]

KEYWORDS

- Diabetes • Lipids • Nursing • Practice applications

KEY POINTS

- Lipid abnormalities in people with diabetes is a major contributing factor to cardiovascular risk in patients with type 2 diabetes.
- Primary care practitioners are at the forefront of screening, diagnosing, and treating patients with diabetes and abnormal lipids to prevent cardiovascular risks and other comorbid chronic conditions.
- Although low-density lipoprotein cholesterol (LDL-C) may be normal in some cases, there are benefits in lowering high levels of LDL-C in those with diabetes.
- Treatment of abnormal lipids in those with diabetes is effective with combined nonpharmacologic and pharmacologic treatment measures.
- With adequate training, support, and appropriate protocol, nurses are in a unique position to diagnose, treat, educate, and follow those with diabetes and abnormal lipids.

INTRODUCTION

Abnormal lipids, sometimes referred to as diabetes dyslipidemia, is a common condition in patients with diabetes.[1] The abnormal lipid profile of patients with diabetes is usually characterized by high levels of triglycerides (TGs), low levels of high-density lipoprotein cholesterol (HDL-C), and elevated low-density lipoprotein cholesterol (LDL-C) and very low-density lipoprotein (VLDL).[1–3] Diabetes alone is an independent risk factor for atherosclerotic cardiovascular disease (ASCVD),[1] and the chances of having ASCVD especially in those with type 2 diabetes increases with abnormal

This work was supported in part with the facilities and resources of the Houston VA HSR&D Center for Innovations in Quality, Effectiveness and Safety grant (grant CIN-13-413).
[a] Health Sciences Research and Development Center for Innovations in Quality, Effectiveness and Safety, 152, 2002 Holcombe Boulevard, Houston, TX 77030, USA; [b] Michael E. DeBakey Veterans Affairs Medical Center, 152, 2002 Holcombe Boulevard, Houston, TX 77030, USA; [c] Baylor College of Medicine, Houston, TX, USA
* Corresponding author. Health Sciences Research and Development Center for Innovations in Quality, Effectiveness and Safety, 152, 2002 Holcombe Boulevard, Houston, TX 77030.
E-mail address: Ngozi.Mbue@va.gov

lipids.[1] Atherosclerosis can lead to conditions such as acute coronary syndromes (ACS), myocardial infarction, stable or unstable angina, coronary or other arterial revascularization, transient ischemic stroke, peripheral arterial disease, and stroke.[1] These conditions have being recognized in the literature as the leading cause of morbidity and mortality in those patients with diabetes and is associated with high direct and indirect cost in diabetes management.[1] Multiple studies have shown successful management of abnormal lipids in patients with diabetes, using both nonpharmacologic and pharmacologic treatment measures. With the increasing number of patients with abnormal lipids, especially those with type 2 diabetes, health care practitioners, including nurses, have to properly manage patients with diabetes as well as abnormal lipids.[1,4,5]

This article examines the pathophysiology of abnormal lipids, the management of abnormal lipids, and the lipid goals for patients with diabetes. Lastly, this article discusses pharmacologic and nonpharmacologic therapies and the role of primary care providers and nurses in the management of abnormal lipids.

PATHOPHYSIOLOGY OF ABNORMAL LIPIDS IN DIABETES

Abnormalities in lipid metabolism and cardiovascular risks in patients with diabetes have been widely studied. Research shows that abnormal lipids in patients with diabetes are a result of a combination of quantitative, qualitative, and kinetic lipoprotein abnormalities contributing to athrogenic lipid profiles.[6–8] The components of quantitative lipoprotein abnormalities are high TG and low HDL-C levels, whereas VLDL subfraction 1 (VLDL$_1$), small, dense LDLs are the main components of qualitative lipoprotein abnormalities.[6] Moreover, increase in VLDL$_1$ along with reduce breakdown of VLDL and an increase in the breakdown of HDL are associated with kinetic abnormality.[6] Other contributors of abnormal lipid profile include type 2 diabetes, insulin resistance and deficiency, high levels of large TG-rich VLDL and poor clearance of VLDL.[6]

In addition, multiple studies showed the link between the size or density of LDL apolipoprotein (Apo) B and Apo A-I to coronary artery disease (CAD) in those with an abnormal lipid profile.[1,2,8–15] Recent data show that Apo B is a better measure of circulating LDL particle number (LDL-P) concentration and is a more reliable indicator for cardiovascular risk than LDL-C.[16] Apo B is a component of athrogenic particles that include VLDL, intermediate-density lipoprotein, LDL-C, and lipoprotein (a),[16] with each particle containing 1 molecule of Apo B, which makes Apo B one of the most predictive measures of athrogenic lipoprotein particles in circulating blood and recurrent cardiovascular events compared with LDL-C.[16–20]

MANAGEMENT OF ABNORMAL LIPIDS IN PRIMARY CARE

Primary care providers such as medical doctors, doctors of osteopathic medicine, nurse practitioners, and physician assistants, among others are the front-line providers in primary care clinics. They play an important role of screening and diagnosing patients who present for care. For patients with diabetes, obtaining a screening lipid profile, such as total cholesterol (TC), LDL-C, HDL-C, TC, TG, and Apo B,[16] after fasting periods of 9 to 12 hours at the initial medical examination for adults is necessary.[2] If testing for lipids is not done fasting, the values for TC and HDL-C can be considered in making clinical decisions related to abnormal lipids during care, which has to be followed by subsequent LDL-C levels to monitor treatment of abnormal lipids. The American Diabetes Association's 2017 guidelines indicate lipid profile should be done in adult patients with diabetes at diagnosis and every 5 years or more if indicated as well as at the initiation of statin therapy and periodically thereafter. Lifestyle modification should be recommended to all and should be done at the outset,[21] but statin therapy is recommended based on risks.[1,22] Testing for LDL-C should be individualized to monitor for adherence and efficacy of nonpharmacologic treatments and drug therapy.[1] However, frequent LDL-C monitoring should be considered for those with a new onset of ACS.[3] (**Table 1** for specific lipid targets for those with diabetes).

Low-Density Lipoprotein Cholesterol Treatment Goals

Lowering LDL-C levels is the main goal of treatment to prevent or improve macrovascular complications of diabetes, such as stroke and heart attack.[1] The National Cholesterol Education Program Adult Treatment Panel III, and the American Association of Clinical Endocrinologists suggest that LDL-C should be the primary parameter for monitoring cholesterol treatment with set goals for individual patients with diabetes.[2,23,24] Studies show that LDL-C has different sizes and densities, with small dense cholesterol (sdLDL-C) posing the greatest impact on premature cardiovascular disease when compared with LDL-C and TGs alone.[25,26] Small LDL-C particles seem to enter the endothelial barrier more readily than the large LDL-C particles and can cause more damage to the endothelial cells.[27–29] The wall of an artery contains 3 layers: the tunica intima, the tunica media, and the adventitia.[27] The intima and media consist of smooth muscle cells, whereas the outer layer adventitia consists of small blood vessels that supply the larger arteries.[27] An accumulation of LDL-C particles in the arterial intima forms the early step of atherosclerosis (**Table 2**). High numbers of sdLDL are associated with an increased risk for CAD[29] and have been associated with high TG,[30] low HDL-C,[31] insulin resistance,[32] and type 2 diabetes.[27] It has been suggested in the literature that sdLDL concentration might be a better marker of the severity of coronary heart disease than LDL-C.[16–18,26] See **Fig. 1** for the wall of an artery and **Table 2** for specific LDL-C treatment goals.

High-Density Lipoprotein Cholesterol Management Goal

Clinicians should pay close attention to what low HDL-C and high HDL-C might represent with regard to CAD risk for those with diabetes. Low HDL-C is associated with

Table 1
Lipid targets for patients with type 2 diabetes

	High-Risk Patients (T2D, No Other Major Risk, and/or Aged <40 y)	Very-High-Risk Patients (T2D Plus ≥1 Major ASCVD Risk[a] or Established ASCVD)
LDL-C (mg/dL)	<100	<70
Non-HDL-C (mg/dL)	<130	<100
TGs (mg/dL)	<150	<150
TC/HDL-C	<3.5	<3.0
Apo B (mg/dL)	<90	<80
LDL-P (nmol/L)	<1200	<1000

Abbreviation: T2D, type 2 diabetes.
[a] Hypertension, family history of ASCVD, low HDL-C, smoking.
Adapted from Garber AJ, Abrahamson MJ, Barzilay JI et al. Consensus statement by the American Association of Clinical Endocrinologist and American College of Endocrinology on the comprehensive type 2 diabetes management algorithm–2016 executive summary. Endocr Pract 2016;22(1):1–30; and Garber AJ, Abrahamson MJ, Barzilay JI, et al. Consensus statement by the American Association of Clinical Endocrinologists and American College of Endocrinology on the comprehensive type 2 diabetes management algorithm–2017 executive summary. Endocr Pract 2017;23(2):207–38.

Table 2
Coronary artery disease risk categories and low-density lipoprotein cholesterol treatment goals

Risk Category	Risk Factors/10-y Risks	LDL-C Treatment Goals
Very high risk	Established or recent hospitalization for coronary, carotid, PVD, DM, plus 1 or more additional risk factors	<70 mg/dL
High risk	≥2 Risk factors and 10-y risk >20% or CHD risk equivalents including DM with no other risk factors	<100 mg/dL
Moderately high risk	≥2 Risk factors and 10-y risk 10%–20%	<130 mg/dL
Moderate risk	≥ Risk factors and 10-y risk <10%	<130 mg/dL
Low risk	≤1 Risk factor	<160 mg/dL

Note: Use the Framingham risk scoring system to identify those with a 10-year risk.

Abbreviations: CHD, coronary heart disease; DM, diabetes mellitus; PVD, peripheral vascular disease.

Adapted from Jellinger PS, Smith DA, Mehta AE, et al. Consensus statement by the American Association of Clinical Endocrinologists task force for the Management of Dyslipidemia and Prevention of Atherosclerosis Writing Committee. Endocr Pract 2012;18(1):1–78; and *Courtesy of* National Cancer Institute, Rockville, MD (Seer Training Modules).

hypertriglyceridemia and may act as a synergy with other abnormal lipid profile components, such as LDL-C and TG, to increase the risk of CAD.[2,33] A high HDL-C level greater than 60 mg/dL is an independent negative risk factor for CAD in both men and women.[2] High levels of HDL-C are important in negating the impact of CAD. Research shows that an HDL-C level greater than 60 mg/dL warrants subtracting one risk factor from overall patients' risk factor profile,[2,33] making it important to encourage high levels of HDL-C in patients. Furthermore, every 1.0-mg/dL increase in HDL-C is associated with a 2% decrease in the risk of CAD in men and a 3% decrease in the risk of CAD in women.[2,33] In addition, the ratio of TC or LDL-C to HDL-C is an emerging, clinically important biomarker when considering CAD risk factors.[2,34–38] However, it is not clear if increasing the HDL-C levels independent of other abnormal lipids levels will solely reduce the risk of CAD.[2] It is important to note that abnormalities of HDL-C can be as a result of genetic and environmental factors, with some individuals having greater risk of CAD than others. Although HDL-C is important in monitoring and treating abnormal lipids, LDL-C remains the primary goal of treatment, especially when considering statin therapy for an abnormal lipid

Artery Wall

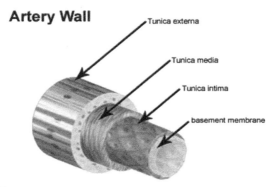

Tunica externa
Tunica media
Tunica intima
basement membrane

Fig. 1. Artery wall.

profile in patients with diabetes,[1,23] though some studies suggest treating to statin intensity as opposed to a certain level of LDL-C[24] (**Table 3** different levels of lipid concentration).

Triglyceride-C Management Goals

Studies show a relationship between high TG and the risk of CAD.[2,39,40] However, information showing TG as an independent risk factor for CAD is lacking.[2,41] It is important to note that studies have shown a relationship between high TG with TC, LDL-C, and HDL-C levels.[2] High TG is said to be, in part, due to other nonlipid risk factors, such as obesity, hypertension, diabetes, and cigarette smoking, among others.[2,42] These important relationships should warrant monitoring TG levels, especially in people with diabetes, as the aforementioned risk factors are also risk factors for CAD.[2,42] Thus, high TG of 200 mg/dL or greater poses a high risk for CAD, beyond the risk of LDL-C alone,[2,43,44] making it absolutely important to monitor and address high levels of TG in those with diabetes to eliminate or delay the risk of CAD[2,43,44] (**Table 4** for TG levels).

PHARMACOLOGIC MANAGEMENT STRATEGIES
Statins (Hydroxymethylglutaryl-Coenzyme A Reductase Inhibitors)

When patients cannot achieve a lipid profile improvement from lifestyle therapies, such as smoking cessation, physical activity, diet modification, and weight loss, pharmacologic therapy should be considered.[45,46] For primary prevention of coronary heart disease, statin therapy has been widely suggested.[22,47,48] Evidence from meta-analyses and random clinical trials suggested using a statin as a first-line drug therapy unless contraindicated; prescribing moderate- to high-intensity doses of statins for qualified patients has been recommended.[45,49–52] Although high-dose statin

Table 3
Optimal/near-optimal, borderline, and high-risk serum lipid concentration

Lipid	Optimal/Near-Optimal Serum Concentration	Borderline Serum Concentration	High-Risk/Very High-Risk Serum Concentration
TC, mg/dL	<200	200–239	≥240
HDL-C, mg/dL	≥60 (neg risk factor)	40–59 (men) 50–59 (women)	<40 men <50 women[b]
LDL-C, mg/dL	<100 optimal (100–129 near-optimal)	130–159	160–189 high ≥190 very high
TG[a], mg/dL	<150	150–199	200–499 high ≥500 very high
Apo B, mg/dL	<90 (patients at risk of CAD, including those with diabetes) <80 (patients with established CAD or diabetes plus ≥1 additional risk factors)		

Abbreviation: Neg, negative.
[a] Both borderline and high-risk values may signify familial combined dyslipidemia or dyslipidemia of diabetes; values greater than 1000 indicate high risk for pancreatitis.
[b] Moderate reductions of high-density lipoprotein cholesterol in women may indicate insulin resistance syndrome.
Adapted from Jellinger PS, Smith DA, Mehta AE, et al. Consensus statement by the American Association of Clinical Endocrinologists" task force for the Management of Dyslipidemia and Prevention of Atherosclerosis Writing Committee. Endocr Pract 2012;18(1):1–78.

Table 4
Classification of elevated triglycerides levels

TG Category	TG Concentration (mg/dL)	Goal
Normal	<150	<150
Borderline-high	150–199	
High	200–499	
Very high	≥500	

Adapted from Jellinger PS, Smith DA, Mehta AE, et al. Consensus statement by the American Association of Clinical Endocrinologists task force for the Management of Dyslipidemia and Prevention of Atherosclerosis Writing Committee. Endocr Pract 2012;18(1):1–78.

therapy can lower LDL-C levels and reduce the risk of ASCVD,[53] it is important to use caution to avoid other risk factors, such as myopathy and liver disorder, linked to using high doses of statins.[45,54,55]

The safety of lipid-lowering drugs, especially statins, has been widely studied. In clinical trials, studies show that nonadherence and discontinuation of lipid-lowering drugs is mostly due to adverse effects, such as increase liver and muscle enzymes, which is estimated to be around 10% to 15%, requiring prompt monitoring of therapies.[46,47,56,57] If therapeutic levels of LDL-C, non–HDL-C, Apo B, or LDL-P is not reached while on a statin, adding other combined drug therapies should be considered.[45]

Fibrates (Peroxisome Proliferator-Activated Receptor-α Agonists)

Fibrates are used to lower high TG levels.[8,58] Fibrates have the additional advantage of increasing HDL-C levels.[8] In clinical practice, the use of fibrates as a monotherapy[58] may result in worse outcomes, especially in patients with diabetes with high cardiovascular risk factors. However, in individuals with diabetes, a combination of statin and fenofibrate therapy has a better outcome of lowering LDL-C and TG and increasing HDL-C levels.[58,59] The use of fibrates is indicated in lowering LDL-C and in reversing the smaller-density LDL phenotype as well.[60–62] Fibrates are well tolerated with fewer adverse effects; however, care should be taken in those with impaired hepatic and renal function.[8]

Niacin

Nicotinic acid (niacin) increases HDL-C levels with fewer effects on TG and LDL-C.[8,63] High doses of niacin have been shown in studies to increase blood glucose levels, especially in individuals with prediabetes and newly diagnosed individuals with diabetes.[8,63] Niacin is well tolerated but commonly causes flushing. To prevent flushing, an aspirin should be taken 30 minutes before taking niacin. Niacin should not be taken with a hot beverage or alcohol.[64]

Bile Acid Sequestrants

Bile acid sequestrants lower hypercholesterolemia.[65] They lower LDL-C levels and can be used as a monotherapy or in combination with statins, fibrates, and/or cholesterol absorption inhibitors.[65] In addition to lowering LDL-C levels, it increases HDL-C levels as well.[2] Research shows that it can also improve blood glucose in those with type 2 diabetes.[65–69] Bile acids have been known to have a high discontinuation rate mostly due to gastrointestinal tract–related adverse effects[2,70]; however, colesevelam is well tolerated when compared with the other bile acids.[2,71,72] For patients with diabetes with high TG, care should be taken, as bile acid has the potential to increase TG levels.[2,72–75]

Cholesterol Absorption Inhibitors

Ezetimibe is the only drug currently available in this family of cholesterol absorption inhibitiors.[2,76,77] Cholesterol absorption inhibitors reduce LDL-C and may also have beneficial effects on Apo B, TG, and HDL-C, especially in combination with statins.[2] Ezetimibe has lower adverse effects and is generally well tolerated; however, care should be taken when administering to patients with decreased hepatic function.[2]

Combination Therapies

When monotherapy is not effective, a combination therapy, such as a statin with a cholesterol absorption inhibitor or a statin with a bile acid sequestrant, a fibrate, or an extended-release niacin, may be warranted based on the patient profile.[22] Of all these combinations, the statin-sequestrant may be the most effective in reducing LDL-C by as much as 70%.[22] Although a statin-fibrate combination can reduce both LDL-C and VLDL-C,[22] it is important to carefully monitor patients on combination therapy for adverse effects that may include muscle pain to high liver enzymes[22] (**Table 5** for all lipid-lowering therapies).

OTHER PHARMACOLOGIC REGIMENS

Other important pharmacologic therapies to be considered for some patients with diabetes include n-3 fatty acids α linolenic acid, eicosapentaenoic acid (EPA), and docosahexaenoic acid (DHA), which have been recognized to prevent and treat cardiovascular disease.[78] Higher doses of DHA and EPA lower TG and its production and represent an alternative to fibrates or nicotinic acid for the treatment of high TG.[22] DHA and EPA are available in capsules of fish oil, and doses of 3 to 12 g/d have been use based on tolerance level. The n- 3 fatty acids can come from foods high in n-3–rich vegetable oils of fatty fish or fish oil supplements.[22]

NONPHARMACOLOGIC STRATEGIES/INTERVENTIONS

Research shows that diet modification, exercise, weight control, and/or smoking cessation are all effective ways to prevent high lipid levels and prevent CAD.[2]

Medical Nutrition Therapy

Studies show diet modification to be an integral part of cholesterol control. Medical nutrition therapy administered and monitored by a registered dietician can be cost-effective and efficacious in reducing LDL-C and TC and improving blood glucose levels.[2,79,80] Adding plant stanol esters has shown to lower TC and LDL-C.[2,81] Plant stanol is found in most fruits, nuts, vegetables, legumes, vegetable oils, and beverages and has shown to reduce LDL-C by 10% to 15% without side effects, especially at a level of 2 to 3 g/d.[81] Individuals with diabetes and high lipids should consume foods high in fiber and low in saturated fat and cholesterol.[82]

Exercise and Weight Control

Exercise, when medically safe, is encouraged as an adjunct to weight control and in the prevention of heart disease.[82] In individuals with diabetes, weight programs that achieve a 500- to 750-kcal/d energy deficit or provide approximately 1200 to 1500 kcal/d for women and approximately 1500 to 1800 kcal/d for men is beneficial in blood glucose control and lipid control.[80] For obese individuals with type 2 diabetes,

Table 5
Lipid-lowering therapies

Medications	Usual Recommended and Start Daily Dose	Dose Range
Statins		
Atorvastatin	10–20 mg	10–80 mg
Fluvastatin	40 mg	20–80 mg
Lovastatin	20 mg	10–80 mg
Pitavastatin	2 mg	2–4 mg
Pravastatin	40 mg	10–80 mg
Rosuvastatin	10 mg	5–40 mg
Simvastatin	20–40 mg	5–80 mg[a]
Fibrates		
Fenofibrate	48–145 mg	48–145 mg
Fenofibric	45–135 mg	45–135 mg
Gemfibrozil	1200 mg	1200 mg
Niacin		
Immediate release	250 mg	250–3000 mg
Extended release	500 mg	500–2000 mg
Bile acid sequestrants		
Cholestyramine	8–16 g	4–24 g
Colestipol	2 g	2–16 g
Colesevelam	3.8 g	3.8–4.5 g
Cholesterol absorption inhibitors		
Ezetimibe	10 mg	10 mg
Combination therapies (single pill)		
Ezetimibe/simvastatin	10/20 mg	10/10–10/80 mg
Extended-release niacin/simvastatin	500/20 mg	500/20–1000/20 mg

Note. Simvastatin, 80 mg, is not approved for therapy unless patients have been on treatment for more than 1 yeat without myopathy.
  [a] Hypertension, family history of ASCVD, low HDL-C, smoking.
  Adapted from Jellinger PS, Smith DA, Mehta AE, et al. Consensus statement by the American Association of Clinical Endocrinologists" task force for the Management of Dyslipidemia and Prevention of Atherosclerosis Writing Committee. Endocr Pract 2012;18(1):1–78.

sustained weight loss of 7% or greater of total body weight is crucial in optimal control of blood glucose and lipid levels.[80]

Smoking Cessation

Smoking cessation improves long-term cardiovascular outcomes.[2,83–86] Smoking is one of the avoidable causes of death in the United States.[87] Studies show macrovascular and microvascular complications are common in smokers who have diabetes compared with the general population.[87] An abnormal lipid profile in smokers with diabetes worsens insulin resistance, thereby leading to further cardiovascular problems.[87] Clinicians should strive to encourage smoking cessation, especially in those with diabetes with elevated levels of abnormal lipids either by encouraging the use of pharmacotherapy or proven behavioral intervention therapies.[87]

ROLE OF NURSES IN THE MANAGEMENT OF ABNORMAL LIPIDS

With the increase of health care needs and an aging population, nurses are more than ever needed to care for the increasing health care needs of patients, especially those with chronic diseases.[88] Providing quality and affordable care will need a team approach that will involve nurse-managed protocols.[88] Nurses are strategically positioned in both primary care, inpatient and in communities to treat, monitor and educate patients in various disease processes, especially in diabetes care.[89] Medical management of chronic conditions consumes appropriately 75% of health care cost in the United States. Patients with diabetes and hyperlipidemia have a high morbidity and mortality rate.[89–91] To decrease the burden, a joint effort is imperative to manage glucose and lipids.

A patient-centered medical home was developed to serve more individuals and improve the care of chronic diseases.[89] Care teams in the medical model home may include registered nurses,[89] who are currently the largest health care workforce and may be important assets alongside other nonphysician clinicians.[89] As the management of diabetes and high cholesterol are mostly carried out in outpatient clinics, with clearly defined protocols and training, nurses can order diagnostic tests, interpret test results, adjust routine medications, and conduct appropriate referrals whenever necessary.[89] Studies show that nurses are a clinically experienced work force and can adhere to treatment protocols in studies that examined pharmacologic therapies for lipid management.[78,89,92,93] In addition, nurse-managed protocols have a consistently positive effect in those with chronic diseases in multiple studies.[89]

SUMMARY

This article provides an overview of the pathophysiology of abnormal lipids in those with diabetes, management of lipids in primary care, and management goals for lipids for patients with diabetes. In addition, discussions of the pharmacologic and nonpharmacologic therapies, the role of primary care providers and nurses in the management of abnormal lipids in those with diabetes.

Lipid abnormalities in people with diabetes are a major contributing factor to cardiovascular risk in patients with type 2 diabetes. Lipid abnormalities include abnormal quantitative, qualitative, and kinetic lipoproteins that are primarily athrogenic. High levels of TG and low levels of HDL-C are common in those with diabetes. Although levels of LDL-C may be normal in some individuals with diabetes, it is beneficial to lower LDL-C in those with high levels of LDL-C. Primary care providers should strive to treat to recommended goals for lipids for those with diabetes. Nurses are now more than ever needed in the management of chronic diseases and especially in managing abnormal lipid levels alongside diabetes care. Nurses are in a unique position to manage patients with an abnormal lipid profile. With adequate training and support, nurses can be a force in helping control the cost of chronic conditions along with the cost of managing abnormal lipids in patients with diabetes.

REFERENCES

1. American Diabetes Association. Standards of medical care in diabetes. Diabetes Care 2017;40(1):S1–135.
2. American Association of Clinical Endocrinologist. Guidelines for management of dyslipidemia and prevention of atherosclerosis. Available at: https://www.ncbi.nlm.nih.gov/pubmed/22522068. Accessed November 20, 2016.

3. Barnett A. Management of lipids in patients with diabetes. Diabetes Obes Metabol 2003;5(1):S3–9.

4. American Association of Clinical Endocrinologist. Guidelines for management of dyslipidemia and prevention of atherosclerosis. Available at: https://www.AACE DYSLIPIDEMIA 2012.pdf. Accessed November 20, 2016.

5. Tressler MC, Greer N, Rector TS, et al. Factors associated with treatment success in veterans with diabetes and hyperlipidemia: a retrospective study. Diabetes Educ 2013;39(5):664–70.

6. Costa J, Borges M, David C, et al. Efficacy of lipid lowering drug treatment for diabetic and non-diabetic patients: meta-analysis of randomized controlled trials. Br Med J 2006;1–10. http://dx.doi.org/10.1136/bmj.38793.468449.AE.

7. Verges B. Pathophysiology of diabetic dyslipidemia: where are we? Diabetologia 2015;58:886–99.

8. Parhofer KG. Pathophysiology of diabetic dyslipidemia: implications for atherogenesis and treatment. Clinical Lipidology 2011;6(4):401–11.

9. Krauss RM. Lipids and lipoproteins in patient with type 2 diabetes. Diabetes Care 2004;27(6):1496–504.

10. Austin MA, King MC, Vranizan KM, et al. Atherogenic lipoprotein phenotype: a proposed genetic marker for coronary heart disease risk. Circulation 1990; 82(2):495–506.

11. Austin MA, Breslow JL, Hennekens CH, et al. Low density lipoprotein subclass patterns and risk of myocardial infarction. JAMA 1988;260(13):1917–21.

12. Campos H, Genest JJ Jr, Blijlevens E, et al. Low density lipoprotein particle size and coronary artery disease. Arterioscler Thromb Vasc Biol 1992;12:187–95.

13. Coresh J, Kwiterovich PO Jr, Smith HH, et al. Association of plasma triglyceride concentration and LDL particle diameter, density, and chemical composition with premature coronary artery disease in men and women. J Lipid Res 1993; 34(10):1687–97.

14. Crouse JR, Parks JS, Schey HM, et al. Studies of low density lipoprotein molecular weight in human beings with coronary artery disease. J Lipid Res 1985;26(5): 566–74.

15. Gardner CD, Fortmann SP, Krauss RM, et al. Association of small low-density lipoprotein particles with the incidence of coronary artery disease in men and women. JAMA 1996;276(11):875–81.

16. Sigurdsson AF. Metabolic syndrome and insulin resistance. Available at: http://www.docsopinion.com/2015/01/29/metabolic-syndrome-insulin-resistance-syndrome/. Accessed December 2, 2016.

17. Contois JH, McConnell JP, Sethi AA. Apolipoprotein B and cardiovascular disease risk: position statement from the AACC Lipoproteins and Vascular Diseases Division Working Group on best practices. Clin Chem 2009;55(3):407–19.

18. Thompson A, Danesh J. Association between apolipoprotein B, apolipoprotein AI, the apolipoprotein B/AI ratio and coronary heart disease: a literature-based meta-analysis of prospective studies. J Intern Med 2006;259:481–92.

19. Shen H, Xu Y, Lu J. Small dense low-density lipoprotein cholesterol was associated with future cardiovascular events in chronic kidney disease patients. BMC Nephrol 2016;17:143–50.

20. Lamarche B, Tchernof A, Moorjani S. Small, dense low-density lipoprotein particles as a predictor of the risk of ischemic heart disease in men. Circulation 1997;95:69–75.

21. Reusch JE, Manson JE. Management of type 2 diabetes in 2017. Getting to goal. JAMA 2017;317(10):1015–6.

22. Daniel MJ. Lipid management in patients with type 2 diabetes. Am Health Drug Benefits 2011;4(5):312–22.

23. St-Pierre A, Cantin B, Dagenais GR, et al. Low density lipoprotein subfractions and the long-term risk of ischemic heart disease in men: 13-year follow-up data from the Quebec Cardiovascular Study. Arterioscler Thromb Vasc Biol 2005;25:553–9.

24. Wu A, Li J. Clinical considerations for lipid target and goal in dyslipidemia control. Chronic Dis Translational Med 2016;2:3–6.

25. Expert Panel on Detection, Evaluation, and Treatment of High Blood Cholesterol in Adults. Executive summary of the Third Report of the National Cholesterol Education Program (NCEP) Expert Panel on Detection, Evaluation, and Treatment of High Blood Cholesterol in Adults (Adults Treatment Panel III). JAMA 2001;285(19):2486–97.

26. Kataoka Y, Andrews J, Puri R, et al. Plaque burden, microstructures and compositions underachieving very low LDL-C levels. Curr Opin Endocrinol Diabetes Obes 2017;24. http://dx.doi.org/10.1D.1D97/MED.0000000000000317.

27. Kikka K, Nakajima K, Shimomura Y, et al. Small dense LDL Cholesterol measured by homogeneous assay in Japanese healthy controls, metabolic syndrome and diabetes patients with or without a fatty liver. Clin Chim Acta 2015;438:70–9.

28. Sigurdsson AF. Low-density lipoprotein (LDL) in atherosclerosis and heart disease. 2016. Available at: https://www.docsopinion.com/2016/01/25/low-density-lipoprotein-in-atherosclerosi-and-heart-disease/. Accessed February 20, 2017.

29. Younis NN, Soran H, Pemberton P. Small dense LDL is more susceptible to glycation than more buoyant LDL in type 2 diabetes. Clin Sci 2013;124:343–9.

30. Coresh J, Kwiterovich PO. Small dense low-density lipoprotein particles and coronary heart disease risk. A clear association with uncertain implications. JAMA 1996;276(11):914–5.

31. Sigurdsson AF. High-triglycerides-how to lower triglycerides. Available at: http://www.docsopinion.com/2016/01/03/high-triglycerides-lower-triglycerides/. Accessed December 2, 2016.

32. Sigurdsson AF. HDL Cholesterol- the "good" cholesterol explained. Available at: https://www.docsopinion.com/2014/08/12/hdl-cholesterol. Accessed December 2, 2016.

33. AHA/ACC Cholesterol treatment guidelines (November, 2013): relevance to patients with diabetes. Available at: https://www.joslin.org/info/summary-new-cholesterol-recommendations-11-15-13.html. Accessed February 22, 2017.

34. Third Report of the National Cholesterol Education Program (NCEP) Expert Panel on Detection, Evaluation and Treatment of High Blood Cholesterol in Adults (Adults Panel III) final report. Circulation 2002;106(25):3143–421.

35. Millian J, Pinto X, Munoz A. Lipoprotein ratios: physiological significance and clinical usefulness in cardiovascular prevention. Vasc Health Risk Manag 2009;5:757–65.

36. Upadhyay RK. Emerging risk biomarkers in cardiovascular diseases and disorders. J Lipids 2015;1–51. http://dx.doi.org/10.1155/2015/971453.

37. Lemieux I, Lamarche B, Couillard C. Total cholesterol/HDL cholesterol ratio vs LDL cholesterol/HDL cholesterol ratio as indices of ischemic heart disease risk in men. Arch Intern Med 2001;161:2685–92.

38. Huang H, Mai W, Liu D. The oxidation ratio of LDL: a predictor for coronary artery disease. IOS Press 2008;24:341–9.

39. Sigurdsson AF. The triglyceride/HDL cholesterol ratio. Available at: https://www.docsopinion.com/2014/07/17/triglyceride-hdl-ratio/. Accessed February 23, 2017.

40. Sarwar N, Danesh J, Eiriksdottir G. Triglycerides and the risk of coronary heart disease 10 158 incident cases among 262 525 participants in 29 western prospective studies. Circulation 2007;115:450–8.

41. Miller M, Stone NJ, Ballantyne C. Triglycerides and cardiovascular disease. A scientific statement from the American Heart Disease. Circulation 2011;123:2292–333.

42. Harchaoui KE, Visser ME, Kastelein JJ. Triglycerides and cardiovascular risk. Curr Cardiol Rev 2009;5(3):216–22.

43. American College of Cardiology. CardioSmart. Very high triglycerides. Available at: https://www.cardiosmart.org/vhtg. Accessed February 23, 2017.

44. Gotto AM. Low high-density lipoprotein cholesterol as a risk factor in coronary heart disease. A working group report. Circulation 2001;103:2213–8.

45. Grisanti R. Prevent a heart attack: know your ratio? Available at: https://www.functionalmedicineuniversity.com/public/796cfm. Accessed February 23, 2017.

46. Consensus statement by the American Association of Clinical Endocrinologists and American College of Endocrinology on the Comprehensive type 2 diabetes management algorithm-2016 executive summary. Available at: https://www.diabetesd.net/wp-content/uploads/2015/06/aace-2016-t2-algorithm.pdf. Accessed February 24, 2017.

47. Shepherd J, Blauw GJ, Murphy MB. Pravastatin in elderly individuals at risk of vascular disease (PROSPER): a randomised controlled trial. Lancet 2002;360(9346):1623–30.

48. Thompson PD. What to believe and do about statin-associated adverse effects. JAMA 2016;316(19):1970.

49. Snow V, Aronson MD, Hornbake ER. Lipid control in the management of type 2 diabetes mellitus: a clinical practice guideline form the American College of Physicians. Ann Intern Med 2004;140:644–9.

50. Colhoun HM, Betteridge DJ, Durrington PN, et al. Primary prevention of cardiovascular disease with atorvastatin in type 2 diabetes in the Collaborative Atorvastatin Diabetes Study (CARDS): multicentre randomised placebo-controlled trial. Lancet 2004;364:685–96.

51. Knopp RH, d'Emden M, Smilde JG, et al. Efficacy and safety of atorvastatin in the prevention of cardiovascular end points in subjects with type 2 diabetes: the Atorvastatin Study for Prevention of Coronary Heart Disease Endpoints in Non-insulin-dependent diabetes mellitus (ASPEN). Diabetes Care 2006;29:1478–85.

52. Cholesterol Treatment Trialists' (CTT) Collaboration, Baigent C, Blackwell L, Emberson J, et al. Efficacy and safety of more intensive lowering of LDL cholesterol: a meta-analysis of data from 170,000 participants in 26 randomised trials. Lancet 2010;376:1670–81.

53. Cholesterol Treatment Trialists' (CTT) Collaborators, Kearney PM, Blackwell L, Collins R, et al. Efficacy of cholesterol-lowering therapy in 18,686 people with diabetes in 14 randomised trials of statins: a meta-analysis. Lancet 2008;371:117–25.

54. Shepherd J, Barter P, Carmena R, et al. Effect of lowering LDL cholesterol substantially below currently recommended levels in patients with coronary heart disease and diabetes: the Treating to New Targets (TNT) study. Diabetes Care 2006;29:1220–6.

55. Cannon CP, Steinberg BA, Murphy SA, et al. Meta-analysis of cardiovascular outcomes trials comparing intensive versus moderate statin therapy. J Am Coll Cardiol 2006;48:438–45.

56. Bruckert E, Hayem G, Dejager S, et al. Mild to moderate muscular symptoms with high-dosage statin therapy in hyperlipidemic patients—the PRIMO study. Cardiovasc Drugs Ther 2005;19:403–14.

57. MRC/BHF Heart Protection Study of cholesterol lowering with simvastatin in 20,536 high-risk individuals: a randomised placebo-controlled trial. Lancet 2002;360(9326):7–22.

58. US Preventive Services Task Force Recommendation Statement. Statin use for the primary prevention of cardiovascular disease in adults. JAMA 2016; 316(19):1997–2007.

59. Roussel R, Chaignot C, Weill A. Use of fibrates monotherapy in people with diabetes and high cardiovascular risk in primary care: a French nationwide cohort study based on national administrative databases. PLoS One 2015;10(6): e0137733.

60. Athyros VG, Papagergiou AA, Athyrou VV. Atorvastatin and micronized fenofibrate alone and in combination in type 2 diabetes with combined hyperlipidemia. Diabetes Care 2002;25:1198–202.

61. Frost RJ, Otto C, Geiss HC. Effects of atorvastatin versus fenofibrate on lipoprotein profiles, low-density lipoprotein subfraction distribution, and hemorheologic parameters in type 2 diabetes mellitus with mixed hyperlipoproteinemia. Am J Cardiol 2001;87:44–8.

62. Guerin M, Le Goff W, Frisdal E. Action of ciprofibrate in type IIb hyperlipoproteinemia: modulation of the athrogenic lipoprotein phenotype and stimulation of high-density lipoprotein-mediated cellular cholesterol efflux. J Clin Endocrinol Metab 2003;88:3738–46.

63. Shepherd J. Mechanism of action of fibrates. Postgrad Med J 1993;69(1):s34–41.

64. Oberwittler H, Baccara-Dinet M. Clinical evidence for use of acetyl salicylic acid in control of flushing related to nicotinic acid. Int J Clin Pract 2006;60(6):707–15.

65. Kamanna VS, Kashyap ML. Mechanism of action of niacin on lipoprotein metabolism. Curr Atheroscler Rep 2000;2:36–46.

66. Handelsman Y. Role of bile acid sequestrants in the treatment of type 2 diabetes. Diabetes Care 2011;34(2):s244–50.

67. Garg A, Grundy SM. Cholestyramine therapy for dyslipidemia in non-insulin-dependent diabetes mellitus: a short-term, double-blind, crossover trial. Ann Intern Med 1994;121:416–22.

68. Kondo K, Kadowaki T. Colestilan monotherapy significantly improves glycaemic control and LDL cholesterol levels in patients with type 2 diabetes: a randomized double-blind placebo-controlled study. Diabetes Obes Metab 2010;12:246–51.

69. Suzuki T, Oba K, Futami S, et al. Blood glucose-lowering activity of colestimide in patients with 2 diabetes and hypercholesterolemia: a case-control study comparing colestimide with acarbose. J Nippon Med Sch 2006;73:277–84.

70. Zieve FJ, Kalin MF, Schwartz SL, et al. Results of the glucose-lowering effect of WelChol Study (GLOWS): a randomized, double-blind, placebo-controlled pilot study evaluating the effect of colesevelam hydrochloride on glycemic control in subjects with type 2 diabetes. Clin Ther 2007;29:74–83.

71. Staels B, Fonseca V. Bile acids and metabolic regulation. Mechanisms and chemical responses to bile sequestration. Diabetes Care 2009;32(2):S245.

72. Insull W, Toth P, Mullican W, et al. Effectiveness of colesevelam hydrochloride in decreasing LDL cholesterol in patients with primary hypercholesterolemia: a 24-week randomized controlled trial. Mayo Clin Proc 2001;76:971–82.

73. Davidson MH, Dillon MA, Gordon B, et al. Colesevelam hydrochloride (cholestagel): a new, potent bile acid sequestrant associated with a low incidence of gastrointestinal side effects. Arch Intern Med 1999;159:1893–900.

74. Ma H, Patti ME. Bile acids, obesity and the metabolic syndrome. Best Pract Res Clin Gastroenterol 2014;28(4):573–83.

75. Herrema H, Meissner M, van Dijk TH. Bile salt sequestration induces hepatic de novo lipogenesis through farnesoid X receptor- and liver X receptor α-controlled metabolic pathways in mice. Hepatology 2009;51(3):806–16.

76. Campbell A. Diabetes medicine: bile acid sequestrants and dopamine receptor agonists. Available at: https://www.diabetesselfmanagement.com/blog/diabetes-mdicine-bile-acid-sequestrants-and-dopamine-receptor-agonists/. Accessed February 28, 2017.

77. Gupta EK, Ito MK. Ezetimibe: the first in a novel class of selective cholesterol-absorption inhibitors. Heart Dis 2002;4(6):399–409.

78. Tshiananga JK, Kocher S, Weber C. The effect of nurse-led diabetes self-management education on glycosylated hemoglobin and cardiovascular risk factors: a meta-analysis. Diabetes Educ 2012;38(1):108–23.

79. Ge L, Wang J, Qi W. The cholesterol absorption inhibitor ezetimibe acts by blocking the sterol-induced internalization of NPC1L1. Cell Metab 2008;7:508–19.

80. Probstfield JL. How cost-effective are new preventive strategies for cardiovascular disease? Am J Cardiol 2003;91:22G–7G.

81. Delahanty LM, Sonnenberg LM, Hayden D, et al. Clinical and cost outcomes of medical nutrition therapy for hypercholesterolemia: a controlled trial. J Am Diet Assoc 2001;101:1012–23.

82. Nguyen TT. The cholesterol-lowering action of plant stanol esters. J Nutr 1999; 129:2109–12.

83. Functional foods fact sheet: plant stanols and sterols. Available at: https://www.foodinsight.org/functional_Foods_Fact_Sheet_Plant_Stanols_and_Sterols. Accessed February 28, 2017.

84. Elixhauser A. The costs of smoking and the cost effectiveness of smoking-cessation programs. J Public Health Policy 1990;11:218–37.

85. Franco OH, der Kinderen AJ, De Laet C, et al. Primary prevention of cardiovascular disease: cost-effectiveness comparison. Int J Technol Assess Health Care 2007;23:71–9.

86. Howard P, Knight C, Boler A, et al. Cost-utility analysis of varenicline versus existing smoking cessation strategies using the BENESCO simulation model: application to a population of US adult smokers. Pharmacoeconomics 2008;26: 497–511.

87. American Diabetes Association. Standards of medical care in diabetes. Diabetes Care 2017;40(1):S1–136.

88. Sheman JJ. The impact of smoking and quitting smoking on patients with diabetes. Diabetes Spectr 2005;18(4):202–8.

89. Shaw RJ, McDuffie JR, Hendrix CC. Effects of nurse-managed protocols in the outpatient management of adults with chronic conditions. Ann Intern Med 2014;16(2):113–22.

90. Bancroft E. How advances in genomics are changing patient care. Nurs Clin North Am 2013;48(2013):557–69.

91. Harris JR, Wallace RB. The Institute of Medicine's new release report on living well with chronic illness. Prev Chronic Dis 2012;9:E148. Available at: https://www.medscape.com/viewarticle/771896. Accessed February 28, 2017.

92. Kung HC, Hoyert DL, Xu J, et al. Deaths: final data for 2005. Natl Vital Stat Rep 2008;56(10):1–20.

93. Halcomb EJ, Davidson PM, Salamonson Y. Nurse in Australian general practice: implications for chronic disease management. J Clin Nurs 2008;17(5A):5–15.

Review of 2017 Diabetes Standards of Care

Kate Crawford, RN, MSN, ANP-C, BC-ADM

KEYWORDS

- Type 1 diabetes • Type 2 diabetes • Prediabetes • Gestational diabetes

KEY POINTS

- Diabetes is one of the most prevalent chronic disorders encountered by health care providers across all specialties and practice settings.
- Diabetes is a complex medical condition that is most effectively treated by knowledgeable providers delivering evidence-based care.
- Multidisciplinary teams using a patient-centered approach that respects patients' preferences and beliefs optimize outcomes.
- Clinical guidelines can assist providers in delivering comprehensive, evidence-based care to promote health and minimize complications.

INTRODUCTION

Diabetes mellitus is a group of complex metabolic disorders characterized by deficient insulin secretion, impaired insulin action, or a combination of both resulting in hyperglycemia. It is a chronic medical condition that requires comprehensive risk-reduction strategies and evidence-based care. This article discusses the current diabetes treatment recommendations for patients with type 1 diabetes (T1DM), type 2 diabetes (T2DM), gestational diabetes (GDM), and prediabetes.

It has been reported that the number of persons with diabetes and prediabetes in the United States is reaching epidemic proportions. In 2014, the Centers for Disease Control and Prevention (CDC) reported diabetes mellitus (DM) affected 29.1 million Americans, or 9.3% of the population.[1] In 2012, approximately 37% of persons older than 20 years were classified as having prediabetes.[1] Outpatient physician visits for diabetes increased 20% from 2005 to 2010.[2] In the acute care setting, 11.5% of all hospitalized patients in 2010 had a diagnosis of diabetes, and diabetes was the second most frequently noted condition on hospital discharge.[3]

Diabetes is a significant source of morbidity and mortality. Compared with adults who do not have diabetes, persons with diabetes are at greater risk for complications and are[1]

Disclosure Statement: There are no commercial or financial conflicts of interest.
North Texas Endocrine Center, 9301 North Central Expressway, Tower II, Suite 570, Dallas, TX 75231, USA
E-mail address: Kate.crawford@aya.yale.edu

- 1.7 times more likely to die of cardiovascular disease
- 1.8 times as likely to have a myocardial infarction
- 1.5 times as likely to have a cerebrovascular accident (CVA)

In 2012, the CDC estimated the total cost of diabetes in the United States to be $245 billion and noted that average medical expenditures for individuals with diabetes to be 2.3 times higher than of persons without the disease.[1]

It is clear given the high prevalence of diabetes and frequency with which patients with diabetes access medical care, that diabetes is a disorder that health care providers will encounter regardless of specialty or area of practice. It is therefore imperative that health care providers are familiar with current guidelines for best practices to promote health and minimize complications.

SUMMARY OF GUIDELINES

Organizations such as the American Diabetes Association (ADA) and the American Association of Clinical Endocrinologists (AACE) issue clinical guidelines that provide recommendations for screening, diagnostic criteria, therapeutic interventions, lifestyle interventions, pharmacology, glycemic goals, A1C targets, and microvascular/macrovascular risk management for persons with diabetes. This article summarizes these recommendations.

PROMOTING HEALTH AND REDUCING DISPARITIES

In 2016, the ADA published a new position statement highlighting the importance of psychosocial needs in the treatment of people with diabetes.[4] They describe tools for assessing patients' environmental, social, behavioral, and emotional influences. The current 2017 guidelines were updated to incorporate the psychosocial needs of the patient across all aspects of care.

In keeping with the new emphasis on the importance of psychosocial needs, the ADA devoted a section of the guidelines to promoting health and reducing disparities in populations. They recommend using the Chronic Care Model (CCM) as a means to remedy some barriers to care that stem from suboptimal delivery systems. Fundamental to the CCM is the concept of a patient empowered to make his or her own self-management decisions and a redefining of the roles of the health care provider from a solitary provider to one practicing in a collaborative, multidisciplinary team.[5]

The CCM is composed of 6 core elements and can be used to address the needs of patients with chronic disease (**Box 1**).

CLASSIFICATION OF DIABETES MELLITUS

Diabetes is not one disease, but rather can be classified into several general categories:

Type 1 Diabetes (T1DM):

- Autoimmune beta cell destruction and absolute insulin deficiency. Presence of autoantibodies

Type 2 diabetes (T2DM):

- Progressive loss of beta cell function and insulin resistance

Gestational diabetes (GDM):

- New-onset diabetes occurring in the second or third trimester

> **Box 1**
> **Chronic care model core elements**
>
> - Optimize team and provider behavior
>   - Team *includes* the patient
>   - Focus on prevention, goal setting, identify and address barriers, integrate evidence-based guidelines, solicit feedback
>   - Incorporate care management teams: nurses, certified diabetes educators, dieticians, pharmacists
> - Empower self-management
>   - Encourage lifestyle changes: healthy eating, physical activity, weight management, tobacco cessation, stress management
>   - Disease self-management: taking medications appropriately, monitoring glucose, blood pressure
>   - Prevent complications: self-foot examinations, dental and ophthalmologic care, immunizations
>   - Identify self-management challenges and assist with goal setting
> - Improve the care system
>   - Use evidence-based guidelines, teams, track adherence at a system level, electronic medical record tools, assess/address psychosocial issues
> - Clinical information systems
>   - Use registries for patient-specific/population-based data
> - Community resources
>   - Identify/develop resources that support healthy choices
> - Health systems
>   - Quality-oriented culture
>
> *Data from* American Diabetes Association. Standards of medical care in diabetes 2017. Diabetes Care 2017;40(Suppl 1):S1–135.

There are many other causes of diabetes, such as monogenic syndromes, exocrine pancreatic dysfunction, and drug/chemical-induced diabetes; however, they are not discussed in this article.

Regardless of etiology, all forms of diabetes are characterized by hyperglycemia.

SCREENING FOR DIABETES, PREDIABETES, AND GESTATIONAL DIABETES

In 2012, approximately 27% of people with diabetes were unaware they had the disease.[1] Given the great cost of diabetes in terms of morbidity and mortality, it is crucial that health care providers understand current guidelines for screening and diagnostic criteria to identify those individuals at risk for or with diabetes.

Screening: Prediabetes

Prediabetes is not a distinct disease but signifies increased risk for the development of diabetes and cardiovascular disease.[5] Patients with glucose values that do not meet the diagnostic criteria for diabetes but are above the normal threshold are described as having prediabetes. Patients with prediabetes exhibit impaired fasting glucose (IFG) and/or impaired glucose tolerance (IGT) and elevated A1C.

It is important that these patients are identified, as it has been estimated that 25% to 50% of patients with IGT and IFG will develop frank diabetes within 5 years.[6]

The ADA and AACE agree on glycemic thresholds for identifying IFG and IGT; however, the AACE criteria for identifying prediabetes is lower than the ADA when using A1C (**Table 1**).[5,7]

Table 1
Glycemic criteria indicating increased diabetes risk (prediabetes)

Organization	IFG, mg/dL	IGT, mg/dL	A1C, %
ADA	100–125	140–199	5.7–6.4
AACE	100–125	140–199	5.5–6.4

Abbreviations: AACE, American Association of Clinical Endocrinologists; ADA, American Diabetes Association; IFG, impaired fasting glucose; IGT, impaired glucose tolerance.

Data from American Diabetes Association. Standards of medical care in diabetes 2017. Diabetes Care 2017;40(Suppl 1):S1–135; and American Association of Clinical Endocrinologists. Diagnosis of type 2 diabetes mellitus. Available at: http://outpatient.aace.com/type-2-diabetes/diagnosis-of-type2-diabetes-mellitus. Accessed May 1, 2017.

Screening: Diabetes and Prediabetes in Adults

Asymptomatic adults who meet the following criteria should be screened for diabetes and prediabetes.[5]

- Body mass index (BMI) greater than 25 kg/m^2 or greater than 23 kg/m^2 in Asian individuals *AND* 1 or more of the following risks:
  - A1C >5.7, IGT or IFG
  - First-degree relative with diabetes
  - High-risk racial/ethnic group
    - African American, Native American, Latino, Asian American, Pacific Islander individual
  - Women with GDM history
  - Women with polycystic ovarian syndrome (PCOS)
  - Cardiovascular disease (CVD)
  - Blood pressure greater than 140/90 or treated for hypertension
  - High-density lipoprotein (HDL) less than 35 mg/dL and/or triglycerides greater than 250 mg/dL
  - Sedentary lifestyle
  - Markers of insulin resistance
    - Severe obesity
    - Acanthosis nigricans
- All patients older than 45
- Retesting
  - If results are normal; repeat every 3 years
  - If prediabetes; repeat yearly
  - Repeat more frequently if risks change, for example, develop CVD

Screening: Children and Adolescents with Type 2 Diabetes Mellitus

Although once considered rare, the incidence of T2DM in children and adolescents has risen dramatically.[5] Asymptomatic children (<18 years old) that meet the following criteria should be screened for diabetes and prediabetes[5]:

- BMI
  - Greater than 85th % for age and sex
  - Greater than 85th % weight for height
  - Weight greater than 120% of ideal for height
- AND 2 additional risks:
  - First-degree or second-degree relative with type 2 diabetes
  - High-risk racial/ethnic group

- African American, Native American, Latino, Asian American, Pacific Islander individual
  - Signs of insulin resistance
    - Acanthosis nigricans, hypertension (HTN), dyslipidemia, PCOS, small for gestational age/birth weight
  - Maternal diabetes or GDM
- At age 10 or onset of puberty if <10
- Retest every 3 years

Screening: Type 1 Diabetes Mellitus

Routine screening for T1DM with antibodies in the general population is not currently recommended; however, screening with autoantibodies is appropriate in research trials or in first-degree family members of newly diagnosed patients.[5]

Screening: Gestational Diabetes

Uncontrolled hyperglycemia poses risks to both mother and fetus.[5] It is therefore important to screen for alterations in glucose metabolism to prevent serious complications. GDM was previously defined as any degree of glucose intolerance first recognized in pregnancy, regardless if the condition predated or continued after the pregnancy.[8,9] Current guidelines recognize the increased prevalence of T2DM and differentiate GDM from preexisting diabetes as diabetes that is first diagnosed in the second or third trimester and is not preexisting T1DM or T2DM.[5] The ADA recommends testing women with risk factors for T2DM (see section above: Screening: Diabetes and Prediabetes in Adults) at the first prenatal visit. When diagnosed in the first trimester, they are diagnosed with T2DM (or rarely T1DM), not GDM. In women without risk factors or a previous diagnosis of diabetes, screening should take place at 24 to 28 weeks gestation.

Screening can be conducted in 1 of 2 ways by using an oral glucose tolerance test (OGTT):

- One-step process
  - 75 g OGTT
  - Fasting
    - 8 hours before test
  - Glucose measurement
    - Fasting
    - One hour after ingestion
    - Two hours after ingestion
  - Diagnostic
    - One value above threshold
      - Fasting: ≥ 92
      - 1 hour: ≥ 180
      - 2 hour: ≥ 153
- Two-step process
  - 50 g OGTT
  - Fasting
    - Not necessary
  - Glucose measurement
    - One hour after ingestion
  - Diagnostic
    - Value above

- Greater than 130
- Greater than 135 or $\geq$140
  - ○ Recommended by American Congress of Obstetricians and Gynecologists (ACOG)
    - If positive
      - Proceed to 100 g OGTT (see **Table 7**)

Table 2 compares the 1-step and 2-step screening methods. Diagnostic criteria are discussed further in the section on diagnosing GDM.

The ADA does not endorse a preferred method of screening; however, ACOG recommends using the 2-step approach.[5] Some providers prefer to use the 2-step process, as the initial 50-g screen does not require the patient to be fasting, requires only 1 venipuncture, and is less time-consuming. A1C is not recommended as a screening tool for GDM.

Women with GDM should be rescreened at 4 to 12 weeks after delivery for persistent hyperglycemia by using a 75 g OGTT and nonpregnancy diagnostic criteria (see **Table 4**). Women with GDM should have lifelong diabetes screening at minimum every 3 years, as they are at greater risk for developing diabetes.[5]

DIAGNOSIS
Diagnosis: Diabetes

Diabetes can be diagnosed using various laboratory tests, including the following:

- Fasting plasma glucose (FPG): no intake for 8 hours
- 2-hour plasma glucose after ingestion of 75 g anhydrous oral glucose (OGTT)
- Hemoglobin A1C

The most sensitive test for diagnosing diabetes is the 2-hour OGTT[5]; however, this may be difficult to administer due to time constraints, and like the FPG, requires that the patient has been fasting for 8 hours. A1C testing is convenient and does not require fasting; however, it can be less accurate in persons of certain races, those with hemoglobinopathies, and anemias. See **Table 3** for a comparison of the diagnostic tests for diabetes.

The ADA considers any of the 3 testing methods appropriate for diagnosing diabetes[5]; however, AACE recommends using FPG or OGTT for diagnosis and A1C as a screening tool.[7] Both associations agree on the glycemic thresholds for diagnosing diabetes (**Table 4**).

Table 2 Gestational diabetes mellitus screening comparison		
	One-Step	**Two-Step**
Carbohydrate, g	75	50 Proceed to 100 if positive
Fasting	Yes	No
Venipunctures	3	1
Time for testing, h	2	1
Glycemic threshold	Fasting: $\geq$92 One hour: $\geq$180 Two hour: $\geq$153	$\geq$130 $\geq$135[a] $\geq$140[a]

[a] American Congress of Obstetricians and Gynecologists criteria.

Data from American Diabetes Association. Standards of medical care in diabetes 2017. Diabetes Care 2017;40(Suppl 1):S1–135.

Table 3
Comparison of diagnostic tests for diabetes

	FPG	75-g OGTT	A1C
Diagnostic for ADA	Yes	Yes	Yes
Diagnostic for AACE	Yes	Yes	Not preferred
8 h fasting	Yes	Yes	No
Special considerations	No	No	Yes
Use with Children/Adolescents DM2	Yes	Yes	Likely yes
Use with Children/adolescents DM1	Yes	Yes	No
Easily available	Yes	Maybe	Maybe

Abbreviations: AACE, American Association of Clinical Endocrinologists; ADA, American Diabetes Association; DM1, diabetes mellitus type 1; DM2, diabetes mellitus type 2; FPG, fasting plasma glucose; OGTT, oral glucose tolerance test.
Data from American Diabetes Association. Standards of medical care in diabetes 2017. Diabetes Care: 2017;40(Suppl 1):S1–135; and American Association of Clinical Endocrinologists. Diagnosis of type 2 diabetes mellitus. Available at: http://outpatient.aace.com/type-2-diabetes/diagnosis-of-type2-diabetes-mellitus. Accessed May 1, 2017.

Glycemic values for patients without diabetes, prediabetes, and diabetes are outlined in **Table 5**.

In the absence of undisputed clinical findings of diabetes (Diabetic ketoacidosis [DKA], Hyperglycemic hyperosmolar nonketotic coma [HHNK], or polyuria, polydipsia, polyphagia with a random plasma glucose >200), testing must be confirmed, preferably repeating the same test. If the same test is repeated and both values are above the diagnostic threshold, the diagnosis is confirmed. If 2 different tests are ordered; for example, FPG and A1C, and only 1 test is above the threshold, the test that is above the threshold should be repeated.[5]

Diagnosis: Type 1 Diabetes Mellitus

Type 1 diabetes is an autoimmune process by which pancreatic beta cells are destroyed and is diagnosed, in addition to glycemic criteria (see **Table 4**), by the presence of 1 or more of the following autoimmune markers[5]:

- Islet cell autoantibodies
- GAD 65 autoantibodies
- Insulin autoantibodies
- Tyrosine phosphatase IA-2, IA-2beta and ZnT8 autoantibodies

Table 4
Criteria for diagnosing diabetes in nonpregnant adults

Test	Result
Fasting plasma glucose	≥126 mg/dL
75-g oral glucose tolerance test	≥200 mg/dL
A1C	≥6.5%
Random plasma glucose	≥200 + symptoms

Data from American Diabetes Association. Standards of medical care in diabetes 2017. Diabetes Care 2017;40(Suppl 1):S1–135.

Table 5
Normal, prediabetes, and diabetes mellitus glycemic values

	Normal	Prediabetes	Diabetes
Fasting glucose	<99	100–125	≥126
Postprandial	≤139	140–199	≥200
A1C	ADA: ≤5.6 AACE: ≤5.4	ADA: 5.7–6.4 AACE: 5.5–6.4	≥6.5
Random	—	—	≥200 + symptoms

Abbreviations: AACE, American Association of Clinical Endocrinologists; ADA, American Diabetes Association.

Data from American Diabetes Association. Standards of medical care in diabetes 2017. Diabetes Care 2017;40(Suppl 1):S1–135, and American Association of Clinical Endocrinologists. Diagnosis of type 2 diabetes mellitus. http://outpatient.aace.com/type-2-diabetes/diagnosis-of-type2-diabetes-mellitus. Accessed May 1, 2017.

Both the ADA and AACE recommend blood glucose, rather than A1C, be used for diagnostic purposes in the acute phase of T1DM as A1C may not have had time to reflect the degree of hyperglycemia.[5,7]

Diagnosis: Children

Although A1C is not recommended for diagnosing acute-onset T1DM, the ADA does recommend using A1C for diagnosing T2DM in children and adolescents despite limited data on the validity of its use in pediatrics (see **Table 3**). They note that there are some data to suggest that OGTT and FPG may be more accurate; however, they do not endorse one test over another.[5]

The diagnostic criteria in children and adolescents are the same as for adults (see **Table 4**).

Diagnosis: Gestational Diabetes

The diagnostic criteria for GDM reflects a lack of consensus among various organizations regarding elevated glycemic thresholds in pregnancy. The National Diabetes Data Group (NDDG), ACOG, and the International Association of the Diabetes and Pregnancy Study Groups have all contributed guidelines.[5] The guidelines recommend using either a 1-step or 2-step approach, both of which have been validated as adequately identifying hyperglycemia in pregnancy.[5] The 2-step process includes 2 sets of diagnostic criteria: from the NDDG and Carpenter/Coustan. ACOG does not endorse one set of criteria; however, the ADA states "it would appear advantageous to use the lower diagnostic threshold."[5] See **Tables 6** and **7** for comparisons of the testing methods and diagnostic criteria in GDM.

Table 6
One-step process for diagnosing gestational diabetes

Fasting 8 h	Yes	
Grams of glucose	75	
Value needed to confirm diagnosis	1	
Glucose values	Fasting	≥92
	1 h	≥180
	2 h	≥153

Data from American Diabetes Association. Standards of medical care in diabetes 2017. Diabetes Care 2017;40(Suppl 1): S1–135.

Table 7
Two-step process; 50-g screen, 100-g confirmation

	50 g	100 g	
Fasting	No	Yes	
Values needed for diagnosis	1	2	
Measurement	—	Carpenter/Coustan OR	NDDG
Fasting	N/A	≥95 mg/dL	≥105 mg/dL
1 h	≥130 mg/dL ≥135 mg/dL (ACOG) ≥140 (ACOG) *Proceed to 100 g*	≥180 mg/dL	≥190 mg/dL
2 h	N/A	≥155 mg/dL	≥165 mg/dL
3 h	N/A	≥140 mg/dL	≥145 mg/dL

Abbreviations: ACOG, American Congress of Obstetricians and Gynecologists; N/A, not applicable; NDDG, National Diabetes Data Group.
Data from American Diabetes Association. Standards of medical care in diabetes 2017. Diabetes Care 2017;40(Suppl 1):S1–135.

COMPREHENSIVE MEDICAL EVALUATION AND ASSESSMENT OF COMORBIDITIES

Patients should have a complete medical evaluation at the initial diabetes visit to

- Confirm the diagnosis and type of DM
- Assess for complications and comorbid conditions
- Review prior treatment and risk factor control in established DM
- Formulate plan of care with the patient

The necessary components of a comprehensive medical evaluation are listed as follows[5]:

- Medical history
  - Onset of DM, previous treatment, complementary/alternative medicine use, comorbidities, dental disease, tobacco/substance use, medication use, hypoglycemia, HTN, hyperlipidemia, complications: retinopathy, neuropathy, nephropathy, coronary artery disease, CVA, myocardial infarction (MI), contraception planning
- Physical examination
  - Height, weight, BMI, growth chart (in children)
  - Blood pressure (BP)
  - Funduscopic examination
  - Thyroid
  - Skin examination
  - Comprehensive foot examination
    - Skin, pulses, reflexes, proprioception, vibratory sense, monofilament
- Laboratory tests
  - A1C, lipids, glucose monitoring, liver function, albumin/creatinine, glomerular filtration rate, thyroid-stimulating hormone
- DM self-management behaviors
  - Prior education, barriers such as limited finances, literacy, support
- Nutrition
  - Nutritional status, eating patterns, eating disorders

- Physical activity
  - Type, duration, aerobic, strength
- Psychosocial health
  - Depression, anxiety, diabetes distress
- Immunizations
  - Flu, Hepatitis B
- Sleep
  - Pattern, duration, sleep apnea
- Referrals
  - Smoking cessation
  - Ophthalmology
    - Dilated eye examination
  - Dental
    - Periodontal disease
  - Podiatry
  - Family planning for women
  - Mental health support
  - Diabetes self-management education (DSME)
  - Diabetes self-management support (DSMS)
  - Medical nutrition therapy (MNT)

Routine health maintenance is an important aspect of diabetes care.

Assessment of Comorbidities

In addition to diabetes-related complications, patients should be screened for common comorbid conditions that affect those with diabetes.

Mental Health

Anxiety and depression are common in people diagnosed with diabetes.[10] It has been reported that 25% of patients with diabetes have depressive disorders or increased depressive symptoms.[11] People with mental health issues, such as depression and anxiety, may find it more difficult to engage in self-care behaviors. It is therefore important to screen for depression and anxiety and refer to the appropriate mental health provider as necessary (**Box 2**).

Box 2
Mental health screening

- Depression: all patients with diabetes
  - Annually
    - Especially with history of depression, anxiety
  - On diagnosis with complication(s)
  - On significant change to health status

- Serious mental illness:
  - For patients prescribed atypical antipsychotics
    - Screen for diabetes/prediabetes annually
  - For patients prescribed second-generation antipsychotics
    - Monitor changes in weight, glycemic control

Data from American Diabetes Association. Standards of medical care in diabetes 2017. Diabetes Care 2017;40(Suppl 1):S1–135.

LIFESTYLE MANAGEMENT

Lifestyle management is one of the most important aspects of diabetes care. Comprehensive lifestyle management should include the following components:

- Diabetes Self-Management Education (DSME)
- Diabetes Self-Management Support (DSMS)
- Nutrition therapy
- Physical activity
- Tobacco cessation
- Psychosocial care

Lifestyle interventions should be mutually agreed on by the patient and care team and should be addressed at every visit.

Diabetes Self-Management Education and Support

Diabetes is a complicated disease that requires patients and caregivers to learn many new skills. The goal of DSME and DSMS is to improve self-management, clinical outcomes, health status, and quality of life. DSME and DSMS programs have been shown to improve patient outcomes and reduce costs.[5] It is recommended that all persons with diabetes participate in DSME to obtain knowledge and skills and in DSMS to assist them with implementing behaviors needed to optimize their health. As with all aspects of care, DSME and DSMS need to be patient-focused, respectful, and responsive to the individual's preferences, needs, and values. The need for DSME and DSMS should be evaluated at the following times:

- At diagnosis
- Annually to assess educational, nutritional, and emotional needs
- When new health conditions, limitations, emotional factors, or changes living needs occur
- During transitions in care

DSME was developed to provide education via a flexible, evidence-based curriculum.[12,13] The core components of diabetes self-management education are as follows[12]:

- Diabetes disease process and treatment options
- Incorporating nutritional management into lifestyle
- Incorporating physical activity into lifestyle
- Using medication(s) safely and for maximal effectiveness
- Monitoring blood glucose and other parameters and interpreting and using the results for self-management decision making
- Preventing, detecting, and treating acute complications
- Preventing, detecting, and treating chronic complications
- Developing personal strategies to address psychosocial issues/concerns
- Developing personal strategies to promote health and behavior change

Nutrition Therapy

Altering one's diet and adhering to a food plan can be one of the most challenging aspects of living with diabetes. All patients with diabetes should receive individualized medical nutrition therapy (MNT) provided by a registered dietician. The ADA does not endorse a specific diet, nor does it make specific macronutrient recommendations. See **Box 3** for the general goals of MNT.[5]

Box 3
General goals of medical nutrition therapy

- Promote and support healthful eating by focusing on nutrient-dense choices and appropriate portion sizes to:
  - Achieve/maintain weight goals
  - Achieve individualized glycemic, blood pressure, and lipid targets
  - Delay/prevent complications

- Assess nutritional needs using personal/cultural preferences, health literacy and numeracy, access to healthful foods, willingness and ability to make behavioral changes, and barriers to change

- Use nonjudgmental approach regarding food choices

- Provide tools for developing healthy eating patterns rather than emphasizing individual macronutrients, micronutrients, or single foods

Data from American Diabetes Association. Standards of medical care in diabetes 2017. Diabetes Care 2017;40(Suppl 1):S1–135.

Specific MNT recommendations are as follows[5]:

MNT
- Recommended for all persons with diabetes
  - T1DM and T2DM on flexible insulin programs: instruct in carbohydrate (CHO) counting to determine mealtime insulin; some patients should also use fat/protein counting
- Patients prescribed fixed insulin dosing: CHO intake should be consistent with regard to timing of meals and amount per meal
- Emphasizing portion control and healthy food choices may be more effective for patients
  - With T2DM not on insulin
  - Who have limited health numeracy or literacy
  - Who are elderly and prone to hypoglycemia

Weight loss
- Obese adults with T2DM and prediabetes will benefit from the following:
  - Modest weight loss (5%–7%) via reduced caloric intake
  - Structured programs to assist with weight loss are preferred

Macronutrient Distribution
- No guidelines for distribution of calories among fats, CHOs, and protein
  - Individualize distribution based on the patient's needs
- Variety of diets are acceptable
  - Mediterranean
  - Dietary Approaches to Stop Hypertension (DASH diet)
  - Plant-based
- Avoid sugar-sweetened beverages
- Minimize consumption of added sugars

Carbohydrates (CHOs)
- No guidelines on ideal grams of CHO per day
- CHOs should come from higher fiber and lower glycemic load foods, such as
  - Whole grains
  - Vegetables, fruits
  - Legumes

- Avoid processed "low-fat" or "non-fat" foods with high sugar content
- Patients treated with insulin must couple insulin administration with CHO intake

Protein
- No guidelines regarding ideal protein intake in absence of kidney disease
  - Approximately 15% to 20% of total calories
  - In persons with kidney disease (albuminuria or reduced estimated glomerular filtration rate [eGFR]), no more than 0.8 g/kg body weight per day
- Higher protein intake of approximately 20% to 30% of calories may improve satiety

Fat
- No recommendations regarding ideal fat content
  - Approximately 20% to 35% of total calories
    - Type of fat consumed is more important than total amount; monounsaturated is preferred
  - Mediterranean diet rich in monounsaturated fat may improve glucose metabolism and reduce CVD risk
- Recommend foods rich in omega 3 fatty acids to prevent or treat CVD
  - Fatty fish (eicosapentaenoic acid [EPA] and docosahexaenoic acid [DHA])
  - Nuts and seeds (alpha-linolenic acid [ALA])
  - No evidence to support omega 3 supplements
- Avoid trans fat

Micronutrients and supplements
- No evidence to support supplements in patients without underlying deficiencies; potential safety issues with long-term use of vitamins E and C and carotene
- Patients treated with metformin should be screened for B12 deficiency

Alcohol
- Men: no more than 2 drinks per day
- Women: no more than 1 drink per day
- Alcohol may increase the risk for hypoglycemia for those taking
  - Insulin, insulin secretagogues
  - Provide education regarding delayed hypoglycemia

Sodium
- Limit to less than 2300 mg a day
- May reduce further in HTN

Nonnutritive sweeteners
- Generally safe within acceptable daily intake levels

Weight Management

Weight management is crucial for overweight and obese patient with diabetes. Even modest weight loss of 5% to 7% can delay the progression to T2DM from prediabetes.[14] Ideally, weight loss would be assisted with a structured program that recommends a caloric deficit of 500 to 750 calories per day.

Physical Activity and Exercise

Physical activity and exercise are crucial components of the diabetes management plan. Physical activity is a general term that encompasses all movement, whereas exercise refers to a specific type of activity that is structured and intended to improve physical fitness.[5] Exercise can improve glycemic control, decrease cardiovascular risks, aid with weight reduction, and improve mood. The guidelines were updated to reflect emerging research on the deleterious effects of sedentary lifestyle on health outcomes.

Physical activity and exercise recommendations are detailed in **Box 4**. Special considerations regarding exercise are detailed in **Box 5**.

Box 4
Exercise recommendations for people with diabetes

Children and Adolescents

- Type 1 diabetes (T1DM), type 2 diabetes (T2DM), and prediabetes
  - ≥60 min/d of moderate to vigorous aerobic activity
  - 3 d/wk vigorous muscle/bone-strengthening activity

Adults

- Most adults older than 18 with T1DM and T2DM
  - More than 150 min/wk moderate to vigorous physical activity
    - Spread over 3 d/wk
    - No more than 2 consecutive days without activity
  - 2 to 3 sessions/wk resistance exercises on nonconsecutive days
- Younger or more fit patients
  - 75 min/wk vigorous-intensity or interval training
- All adults (especially T2DM) should decrease sedentary behaviors
  - Prolonged sitting should be interrupted every 30 minutes
- Older adults
  - Incorporate 2 to 3/wk flexibility and balance training
    - Can include yoga and tai chi

Data from American Diabetes Association. Standards of medical care in diabetes 2017. Diabetes Care 2017;40(Suppl 1):S1–135.

Tobacco Cessation

It has been reported that adults with chronic medical conditions are more likely to use tobacco.[15] People who smoke, or who are exposed to second-hand smoke, are at increased risk for premature death, CVD, and microvascular complications.[5] All patients should be assessed for tobacco use and offered referral to cessation programs.

Psychosocial Issues

Psychological issues can impair an individual's ability or desire to perform diabetes self-care and can therefore have serious effects on the patient's health. As with all other aspects of care, psychosocial care needs to be integrated in a collaborative manner that is patient-centered. Providers should use patient-appropriate standardized and validated tools and refer for positive findings. It is recommended that family members and caregivers be included in the assessment process.[5]

Diabetes distress (DD) has been identified as a distinct disorder that is characterized by significant negative psychological reactions related to the emotional burdens and anxieties specific to managing diabetes.[5] The prevalence of DD has been reported to be 18% to 45%,[16] yet only 24% of patients state that their health care teams assess their psychological needs.[5] Patients should be assessed for DD using

---

Box 5
Exercise considerations in diabetes

- Pre-exercise evaluation
  - Routine testing not recommended for asymptomatic patients
  - Patients at high risk for cardiovascular disease should start with brief, low-intensity exercise
  - Assess for the following conditions that may contraindicate exercise or predispose to injury
    - Uncontrolled hypertension
    - Untreated proliferative retinopathy
    - Autonomic or peripheral neuropathy
    - Foot ulcer or Charcot foot
- Hypoglycemia
  - Patients taking insulin or secretagogues
    - Monitor glucose before exercise
    - Carbohydrate snack if pre-exercise glucose is <100
  - Patients not taking insulin or secretagogues
    - Less risk, no preventive measures recommended
- Exercise and diabetes complications
  - Retinopathy
    - Contraindicated with proliferative retinopathy or sever nonproliferative retinopathy
    - Consult with ophthalmology before initiating exercise
  - Peripheral neuropathy
    - Risk for skin breakdown, infection, and Charcot foot due to decreased pain sensation
    - Patients should have evaluation before initiation
    - Wear proper footwear
    - Daily foot examination
  - Autonomic neuropathy
    - Risk for postural hypotension, silent myocardial infarction
    - Increased risk for hypoglycemia
    - Cardiology evaluation before exercise
  - Diabetic kidney disease
    - No restrictions

Data from American Diabetes Association. Standards of medical care in diabetes 2017. Diabetes Care 2017;40(Suppl 1):S1–135.

---

validated measures and, if identified, referred for specific education to address their unique needs.

Current recommendations for psychological care are outlined in **Box 6**.

PREVENTION OR DELAY OF TYPE 2 DIABETES

Please refer to the earlier section for the guidelines regarding screening for prediabetes and T2DM.

There is clear evidence regarding the role of intensive lifestyle intervention in diabetes prevention from the landmark Diabetes Prevention Program (DPP) study.[17] The major goals of the intensive lifestyle intervention were greater than 7% weight loss and 150 minutes of physical activity per week. The DPP reported a 58% reduction in the development of T2DM in patients who received intensive lifestyle interventions.[17] The ADA recommends referring patients with prediabetes to intensive behavioral lifestyle intervention programs modeled after the DPP. Patients should attempt at minimum 7% initial body weight loss and increase physical activity to 150 minutes per week.

Box 6
Psychological care in diabetes

- Screening for psychological issues should occur
  - At diagnosis
  - At every visit
  - When hospitalized
  - When diagnosed with complications
  - If the patient is experiencing issues with glycemic control, quality of life, or self-management
  - At age ≥65 for cognitive impairment and depression

- Use patient-centered validated tools, assess for symptoms of
  - Diabetes distress
  - Depression
  - Anxiety
  - Disordered eating
  - Diminished cognitive capacity

- When to refer for mental health services
  - Impaired self-care despite receiving individualized DMSE
  - Positive screen for depression using validated tool
  - Positive screen for cognitive impairment
  - Positive screen for anxiety or hypoglycemia
  - Symptoms of or suspicion of disordered eating behavior
  - Intentional omission of medication for weight loss
  - Suspicion of serious mental illness
  - In youth and families with
    - Behavioral self-care difficulties
    - Repeated hospitalizations for DKA
    - Significant distress
  - Declining/impaired ability to perform self-care
  - Before undergoing metabolic surgery or after if patient continues to require support

Abbreviation: DMSE, diabetes self management education.
Data from American Diabetes Association. Standards of medical care in diabetes 2017. Diabetes Care 2017;40(Suppl 1):S1–135.

Pharmacologic Intervention in Prediabetes

Several pharmacologic agents (metformin, alpha-glucosidase inhibitors, orlistat, glucagonlike peptide 1 (GLP-1) agonists, and thiazolidinediones) have been shown to decrease the development of diabetes in persons with prediabetes.[5] Of these agents, metformin has the strongest evidence for its use. Metformin was, however, less effective than the intensive lifestyle intervention in the DPP.[5]

The recommendations for pharmacologic intervention in prediabetes are as follows:

- Consider metformin therapy in patient with prediabetes and
  - BMI ≥35 kg/m^2
  - Age younger than 60
  - Women with prior GDM
  - Rising A1C despite lifestyle intervention
  - Possible B12 deficiency with long-term use
    - Increased risk with anemia or peripheral neuropathy
- Screen for modifiable risk factors for CVD
  - HTN
  - Dyslipidemia
- DSME and DSMS
  - To develop and maintain healthy behaviors

GLYCEMIC TARGETS

Self-monitoring of blood glucose (SMBG) allows patients immediate feedback to evaluate their response to therapy and provides data as to whether glycemic targets are being met; it is an essential component of therapy. Patients and providers can also use A1C and continuous glucose monitoring to evaluate glycemic control. SMBG is a useful tool when evaluating response to MNT, exercise, preventing hypoglycemia, and adjusting medications, in particular prandial insulin doses.

The accuracy of SMBG depends on the user. The patient's monitoring technique should be evaluated at regular interval to ensure proper results.

GLUCOSE MONITORING

Patients on intensive insulin regimens, that is, multiple-dose insulin or insulin pump therapy should monitor glucose at the following times:

- Before meals and snacks
- At bedtime
- Occasionally 2 hours postprandially
- Before exercise
- When they suspect hypoglycemia
- After treatment of hypoglycemia
- Before critical tasks, such as driving

Patients Using Basal Insulin or Oral Agents

There is no consensus on the frequency of SMBG in patients not prescribed intensive insulin management.

Continuous Glucose Monitoring

Continuous glucose monitoring (CGM) devices measure interstitial rather than plasma glucose concentrations. SMBG is still necessary for calibration of the device, and depending on the device, for insulin dosing. CGM use is associated with A1C reduction in patients age 25 years or older with T1DM, but not in children or adolescents.[5] CGM may be most beneficial to patients who experience frequent episodes of hypoglycemia or who have hypoglycemia unawareness. CGM use requires education and ongoing evaluation and support.

A1C Guidelines

Hemoglobin A1C reflects average glycemic control over approximately 3 months; however, it is an indirect measure of glycemia and should be used in conjunction with other values, such as SMBG or CGM data to evaluate control. Conditions that affect red blood cell turnover or hemoglobin can also affect A1C. Additionally, as A1C is an average, it does not indicate the extent of glycemic variability or hypoglycemia. The Diabetes Control and Complications Trial[18] demonstrated that improved glycemic control significantly reduced rates of microvascular and neuropathic complications, as well as CVD, in persons with T1DM, whereas the UK Prospective Diabetes Study demonstrated that improved glycemic control significantly reduced rates of microvascular and neuropathic complications and CVD in persons with T2DM.[19] An A1C goal of less than 7% has been shown to reduce microvascular and CV complications of diabetes.[18,19]

A1C recommendations are discussed in **Box 7**.

Box 7
A1C recommendations

Frequency of A1C testing

- Patients meeting goals and stable control
  - Every 6 months
- Patients not meeting goals or recent treatment adjustment
  - Every 3 months
- Special considerations
  - Unstable patients or those intensively managed; for example, pregnant women with T1DM
    - Less than every 3 months based on clinical judgment

A1C goals

- Less than 6.5%
  - AACE recommendation for nonpregnant adults
  - ADA recommendation if can be achieved without hypoglycemia or polypharmacy
  - Consider in patients
    - Short duration of diabetes
    - Type 2 diabetes on metformin or diet alone
    - Younger patients
    - No significant cardiovascular disease
- Less than 7%
  - ADA recommendation for nonpregnant adults
- Less than 8%
  - Appropriate for
    - History of severe hypoglycemia
    - Limited life expectancy
    - Multiple comorbidities
    - Long-standing diabetes in whom the goal is difficult to achieve despite education and intensive medication management

Data from American Diabetes Association. Standards of medical care in diabetes 2017. Diabetes Care 2017;40(Suppl 1):S1–135; and American Association of Clinical Endocrinologists. Diagnosis of type 2 diabetes mellitus. Available at: http://outpatient.aace.com/type-2-diabetes/diagnosis-of-type2-diabetes-mellitus. Accessed May 1, 2017.

A1C and Glycemic Targets

Glycemic targets should be modified based on individual factors, such as age, duration of diabetes, life expectancy, and hypoglycemia history. ADA and AACE glycemic targets in nonpregnant adults are compared in **Table 8**.

Both the ADA and AACE recommend postprandial glucose testing in persons with before-meal glucose values at goal but elevated A1C.

Hypoglycemia

The primary limiting factor in the management diabetes is hypoglycemia. The ADA guidelines were updated to define a glucose value of less than 54 as clinically significant hypoglycemia.[5] Clinically significant hypoglycemia can cause serious injury due to impaired cognition. Severe hypoglycemia can progress to loss of consciousness, seizures, and death if untreated. Because of their diminished ability to recognize symptoms and effectively communicate their needs, elderly patients with diabetes

Table 8
Glycemic targets for nonpregnant adults

	ADA	AACE
A1C: most patients	<7.0%	<6.5%
A1C: ideal if achieved without hypoglycemia	<6.5%	Closer to normal for healthy patients
Fasting/preprandial	80–130 mg/dL	<110 mg/dL
2-h postprandial	<180 mg/dL	<140 mg/dL

Abbreviations: AACE, American Association of Clinical Endocrinologists; ADA, American Diabetes Association.

Data from American Diabetes Association. Standards of medical care in diabetes 2017. Diabetes Care 2017;40(Suppl 1):S1–135; and American Association of Clinical Endocrinologists. Diagnosis of type 2 diabetes mellitus. Available at: http://outpatient.aace.com/type-2-diabetes/diagnosis-of-type2-diabetes-mellitus. Accessed May 1, 2017.

and young children with T1DM are at higher risk for experiencing clinically significant hypoglycemia. **Table 9** displays the new guidelines on the classification of hypoglycemia.

Table 9
Classification of hypoglycemia

Level 1: Glucose Alert Value	Level 2: Clinically Significant	Level 3: Severe
≤70 mg/dL	≤54 mg/dL	No specific value
• Low enough for treatment • Adjust glycemic management	• Serious clinically significant	• Severe cognitive impairment • Requires external assistance

Data from American Diabetes Association. Standards of medical care in diabetes 2017. Diabetes Care 2017;40(Suppl 1):S1–135.

Treatment

Treat with rapid-acting carbohydrate at blood glucose alert value of ≤70 mg/dL.[5] Pure glucose is preferred.

Glucagon

Glucagon injection should be used for those individuals who are unable or unwilling to consume carbohydrates by mouth. Persons caring for someone with hypoglycemia-prone diabetes should be instructed on the indications for glucagon use and injection technique.

Hypoglycemia prevention

Patients should use SMBG and in some cases CGM to assess therapy and monitor for hypoglycemia. Patients should be instructed on recognizing situations that predispose them to hypoglycemia, such as fasting, skipping or delaying meals, exercise, or during sleep. If hypoglycemia can be avoided for several weeks, counterregulatory response and hypoglycemia awareness may improve. Therefore, it may be necessary to relax glycemic targets in patients with 1 or more episodes of clinically significant hypoglycemia to improve hypoglycemia unawareness.[5] The current recommendations for hypoglycemia management are listed in **Box 8.**

Box 8
Hypoglycemia management

- Assess for hypoglycemia
  - At-risk patients at each visit
  - Assess for symptomatic and asymptomatic hypoglycemia
- Treatment
  - Conscious and glucose ≤70
    - Glucose 15 to 20 g
      - Preferred but any carbohydrate containing glucose is ok
    - Retest glucose in 15 minutes
      - Repeat treatment if glucose remains ≤70
    - Once glycemia is normal, eat a meal or snack to prevent recurrence
  - Conscious and glucose less than 54
    - May require glucagon
  - Unconscious
    - Glucagon injection
      - Instruct patient and caregivers, anyone trained may administer injection

Data from American Diabetes Association. Standards of medical care in diabetes 2017. Diabetes Care 2017;40(Suppl 1):S1–135.

OBESITY MANAGEMENT FOR THE TREATMENT OF TYPE 2 DIABETES

It has been reported that obesity management can delay the development of diabetes and prediabetes[20] and is beneficial in the treatment of T2DM.[21] Modest and sustained weight loss has been reported to affect clinically significant reductions in glucose, A1C, and triglycerides.[19] Greater weight loss yields additional benefit, such as reducing BP, raising HDL and lowering low-density lipoprotein (LDL) cholesterol, and reducing medications needed for glycemic, BP, and lipid control.[5]

This section outlines recommendations for dietary, pharmacologic, and surgical interventions for obesity management in T2DM.

Assessment: Obesity

BMI should be calculated at each visit to determine the presence of overweight or obesity and discussed with the patient. Patients identified as overweight or obese should be counseled on their increased risk for CVD and all-cause mortality.[5]

BMI definitions of overweight and obesity are outlined in **Table 10**.

General recommendations for managing obesity and overweight are described in **Box 9**.

Table 10
Body mass index classification

	Asian	Non-Asian	
Underweight	<18.5	<18.5	
Normal	18.5–22.9	18.5–24.9	
Overweight	23.0–26.9	25–29.9	
Obese	≥27.0	Class I	30.0–34.9
		Class II	35.0–39.9
		Class III	>40.0

Data from Hsu WC, Araneta MR, Kanaya AM, et al. BMI cut points to identify at-risk Asian Americans for type 2 diabetes screening. Diabetes Care 2015;38(1):150–8.

> **Box 9**
> **Managing obesity and overweight in T2DM**
>
> - Overweight and obese patients ready to lose weight
>   - Goal greater than 5% weight loss
>   - Benefit with 5% loss
>   - ≥ 7% is optimal
>   - Use diet, physical activity, and behavior therapy
>   - High-intensity interventions ≥16 sessions/6 months
>   - Diet
>   - Individualized
>   - Caloric restriction is more important than protein, fat, and carbohydrate percentages
>   - Goal 500 to 750 kcal/day deficit
>   - 1200 to 1500 kcal/day total for women
>   - 1500 to 1800 kcal/day total for men
>   - Weight maintenance programs
>   - Long-term (≥1 year) programs should be prescribed for patients who achieve short-term goals
>   - Programs should include
>   - Monthly visits
>   - Weekly or more frequently monitoring of weight
>   - Continued reduced calorie diet
>   - Continued physical activity 200 to 300 min/wk
>   - Special circumstances
>   - Specially selected patients may use very low calorie diets (<800 kcal/d) and meal replacements
>   - Short-term (3 months)
>   - Only by trained professionals in medical setting
>   - Requires close monitoring
>   - May achieve greater short-term weight loss (10%–15%)
>
> *Data from* American Diabetes Association. Standards of medical care in diabetes 2017. Diabetes Care 2017;40(Suppl 1):S1–135.

Pharmacotherapy: Obesity

Providers should first examine their choice of glucose-lowering agents when considering pharmacologic treatments for overweight and obese patients with T2DM. Diabetes medications that also result in weight loss (ex. GLP-1, SGLT2) or are weight neutral (ex. DPP IV, biguanides) are preferred. Medications not prescribed for diabetes can also contribute to weight gain. Providers should assess all medications for potential adverse effects on weight and when possible, provide alternatives.

Approved Weight Loss Medications

Currently, the following 5 medications are approved by the Food and Drug Administration (FDA) for long-term use (>few weeks) for weight loss:

- Orilistat
- Lorcaserin
- Phentermine/toperimate
- Naltrexone/buproprion
- Liraglutide

Medications are to be used to assist patients following reduced calorie diets and are not a substitute for lifestyle changes.[5]

Weight loss medication guidelines are discussed in **Box 10**.

Box 10
Weight loss medication guidelines

- Body mass index (BMI) $\geq$27 kg/m^2
  - AND 1 or more obesity-associated comorbid conditions
    - T2DM
    - Hypertension
    - Dyslipidemia
- BMI $\geq$30 kg/m^2
  - In patients desiring weight loss
- Monitoring of efficacy and safety
  - Monthly for first 3 months
  - Discontinue if
    - Response is insufficient
      - Less than 5% weight loss
    - Safety or tolerability issues

Data from American Diabetes Association. Standards of medical care in diabetes 2017. Diabetes Care 2017;40(Suppl 1):S1–135.

Metabolic Surgery

Due to the extent and rapidity of improvement in glycemia and to reinforce the role of surgery in the treatment of T2DM, bariatric surgery is now referred to as metabolic surgery.[5] Metabolic surgery has been shown in numerous randomized controlled clinical trials to achieve superior glycemic control and reduction of CV risk factors in obese adults with T2DM diabetes as compared with other lifestyle and medical interventions.[22]

Recommend bariatric surgery in T2DM in adults with the following:

- BMI $\geq$40 kg/m^2 ($\geq$37.5 kg/m^2 in Asian American individuals)
  - Recommend regardless of glycemic control
  - Recommend regardless of complexity of medication regimen
- BMI 35.0 to 39.9 kg/m^2 (32.5–37.4 kg/m^2 in Asian American individuals)
  - When hyperglycemic despite lifestyle and optimal medical therapy

Consider bariatric surgery in T2DM in adults with the following:

- BMI 30.0 to 34.9 kg/m^2 (27.5–32.4 kg/m^2 in Asian American individuals)
  - If hyperglycemic despite optimal medical control by oral or injectable (including insulin) medications

There are currently no recommendations regarding metabolic surgery in obese patients with T1DM.

PHARMACOLOGY

Diabetes pharmacology is a complicated and wide-ranging topic. This section summarizes the current recommendations.

Pharmacologic Therapy for Type 1 Diabetes Mellitus

As patients with T1DM are absolutely insulin deficient, insulin is the cornerstone of therapy. Please see **Box 11** for a discussion of pharmacology specific to T1DM.

Box 11
T1DM pharmacology

- Insulin
  - Most treated with basal and prandial insulin
  - Can be treated with continuous subcutaneous insulin infusion; ie, pump therapy
  - Basal
  - Prandial
    - Use rapid-acting insulin analogs to reduce risk for hypoglycemia
    - Adjust dosing based on carbohydrate intake, before-meal glucose, and physical exercise
    - May need to incorporate fat and protein counting in addition to carbohydrate counting

- Other agents
  - Amylin analog
    - Delays gastric emptying, blunts secretion of glucagon, and enhances satiety
    - FDA-approved for use in adults with T1DM
    - Can assist with weight loss and reduced insulin doses
  - Pancreas transplant
    - T1DM and
      - Undergoing renal transplant
      - Post renal transplant
      - Recurrent DKA
      - Severe hypoglycemia
  - Investigational agents
    - Metformin
      - May be useful in overweight patients
      - Not currently FDA approved
    - Incretin therapies
      - Glucagonlike peptide (GLP)-1 agonists and dipeptidyl peptidase-4 inhibitors have potential for beta cell protection
      - Not currently FDA approved
    - Sodium-glucose cotransporter 2 inhibitors (SGLT2)
      - Risk for euglycemic diabetic ketoacidosis
      - Not currently FDA approved

Data from American Diabetes Association. Standards of medical care in diabetes 2017. Diabetes Care 2017;40(Suppl 1):S1–135.

Pharmacologic Therapy in Type 2 Diabetes Mellitus

This section discusses the general guidelines for medication use. Please refer to the additional articles in this edition for a detailed review of pharmacological treatment.

Factors to consider when selecting medications include efficacy, hypoglycemia risk, effect on weight, side effects, cost, and patient preferences. All steps of therapy should include lifestyle management. The general medication guidelines for T2DM are outlined in **Box 12**.

Cardiovascular Disease

Atherosclerotic cardiovascular disease (ASCVD) is the leading cause of morbidity and mortality for people with diabetes.[5] HTN and dyslipidemia commonly coexist with diabetes, and along with diabetes are all risks for ASCVD. As such, patients with diabetes should be assessed at minimum once yearly for cardiovascular (CVD) risk factors including HTN, dyslipidemia, tobacco use, family history of premature coronary disease, and albuminuria.[5]

HTN is defined as sustained BP greater than or equal to 140/90 mm Hg.[5] Achieving BP targets less than 140/90 in persons with diabetes has been shown to reduce CHD events, CVA, and improve diabetic kidney disease.[5]

Box 12
General medication guidelines for T2DM

- Monotherapy
  - Metformin is the preferred initial agent
    - Not for use if estimated glomerular filtration rate (eGFR) less than 30
    - Gastrointestinal effects
  - Assess for B12 deficiency
  - If A1C targets not met after 3 months, proceed to dual therapy

- Dual therapy
  - If A1C ≥9%, initiate dual therapy
  - Continue metformin
  - Add
    - Second oral agent
      - Sulfonylurea
      - Thiazolidinediones (TZD)
      - Dipeptidyl peptidase-4 inhibitor
      - SGLT2 inhibitor
    - GLP-1
    - Basal insulin
  - If A1C targets not met after 3 months, proceed to triple therapy

- Triple therapy
  - Continue metformin + agent from dual therapy
  - Add other agent
    - SGLT2 inhibitor
    - GLP-1 receptor agonist
    - Basal insulin

- Insulin considerations
  - A1C ≥10%
  - Consider when hyperglycemia is severe, greater than 300
  - Consider in patients with weight loss
  - Ketosis

- Established atherosclerotic cardiovascular disease (ASCVD)
  - Consider empagliflozin or liraglutide
    - Both shown to reduce cardiovascular and all-cause mortality

- Other drugs
  - May be used in specific situations but are not often used
    - Inhaled insulin
    - Alpha-glucosidase inhibitors
    - Colesevelam
    - Bromocriptine
    - Pramlintide

Data from American Diabetes Association. Standards of medical care in diabetes 2017. Diabetes Care 2017;40(Suppl 1):S1–135.

Hypertension recommendations for patients with diabetes are listed in **Boxes 13 and 14.**

Lipid Management

Persons withT2DM are at increased risk for lipid abnormalities, which contributes to increased risk for ASCVD.[5] The beneficial effects of statin therapy on ASCVD outcomes in people with and without CHD has been well documented.[5]

Current lipid recommendations are discussed in **Box 15:**

The ADA no longer recommends treatment based on specific LDL goals but rather recommends statin intensity based on risk factors and age (**Table 11**).[5]

Box 13
Hypertension recommendations; screening, goals, treatment

- Screening
  - Measure blood pressure at every visit
  - Measure properly
  - Seated position, feet on floor, arm supported at heart level after 5 minutes of rest
  - If elevated, confirm on separate day
- Goals
  - ADA: <140/90
  - AACE: <130/80
    - ADA if high-risk cardiovascular disease (CVD) and can be achieved without significant treatment burden
  - Pregnant with chronic hypertension
    - 120 to 160/80 to 105
- Treatment
  - > 120/90
  - If overweight or obese
    - Weight loss
    - DASH diet
    - Reduce sodium less than 2300 mg/d
    - Increased potassium, dairy, fruit and vegetables
    - Reduced alcohol
      - Less than 2 drinks per day for men, less than 1 drink per day for women
    - Increased physical activity
  - > 140/90
    - Lifestyle intervention
    - Initiate treatment rapidly and adjust quickly to goal
  - >160/100
    - Lifestyle intervention
    - Initiate dual therapy

Data from American Diabetes Association. Standards of medical care in diabetes 2017. Diabetes Care 2017;40(Suppl 1):S1–135; and American Association of Clinical Endocrinologists. Diagnosis of type 2 diabetes mellitus. Available at: http://outpatient.aace.com/type-2-diabetes/diagnosis-of-type2-diabetes-mellitus. Accessed May 1, 2017.

Unlike the ADA, AACE does define specific LDL targets and stratifies risk into 5 categories: low, moderate, high, very high, and extreme.[23]

For specific lipid targets as outlined by AACE, please refer to the AACE/ACE Consensus statement by the American Association of Clinical Endocrinologists and American College of Endocrinology on the comprehensive type 2 diabetes management algorithm-2017 executive summary in *Endocrine Practice*[23]; available at: https://www.aace.com/sites/all/files/diabetes-algorithm-executive-summary.pdf.

ANTIPLATELET AGENTS

Aspirin has been shown to reduce CV morbidity and mortality in patients with a prior history of CVA or MI.[5] It is less clear if aspirin is beneficial for patients without a history of CV events. Aspirin recommendations are outlined in **Box 16**.

CORONARY HEART DISEASE

Recommendations for coronary heart disease screening and treatment are listed in **Box 17**.

Box 14
Hypertension recommendations: medications

- Medications
  - Include classes demonstrated to reduce cardiovascular events
    - Angiotensin-converting enzyme inhibitor (ACEI)/angiotensin receptor blocker (ARB)
      - First choice in diabetes with albuminuria
    - Thiazide diuretics
    - Dihydropyridine calcium channel blockers
    - Consider bedtime dosing for at least 1 medication
  - Urinary albumin-creatinine ratio greater than 300 mg/g creatinine
    - ACEI/ARB
      - At maximum tolerated dose indicated for blood pressure management
      - If unable to tolerate ACE
        - ARB
  - If using ACEI/ARB or diuretic
    - Monitor creatinine, eGFR, and potassium
  - Pregnancy
    - Safe to use
      - Methyldopa
      - Labetolol
      - Hydralazine
      - Carvedilol
      - Clonidine
      - Long-acting nifedipine
    - Do NOT use
      - ACEI/ARB
      - Spironolactone

Data from American Diabetes Association. Standards of medical care in diabetes 2017. Diabetes Care 2017;40(Suppl 1):S1–135.

MICROVASCULAR COMPLICATIONS AND FOOT CARE

Microvascular complications of diabetes include nephropathy, retinopathy, and neuropathy. Screening for and treatment of each of these complications is discussed.

Diabetic Kidney Disease

Chronic kidney disease is diagnosed by the occurrence of increased albumin excretion or albuminuria, reduced eGFR, or other indicators of kidney damage. Diabetic kidney disease (DKD) occurs in 20% to 40% of patients with diabetes and is the leading cause of end-stage renal disease.[24] It has been reported that DKD usually takes 5 to 10 years to develop in T1DM but can be present at diagnosis of T2DM.[5] **Box 18** details the current recommendations for DKD.

Diabetic Retinopathy

Patients with T1DM and T2DM are at increased risk for diabetic retinopathy (DR). Both the duration of the disease and degree of glycemic control strongly contribute to the development of DR. DR has been shown to improve with intensive glycemic control and BP management.[18] Current recommendations regarding DR are listed in **Box 19**.

Neuropathy

Diabetic neuropathies are a group of disorders with widely variable presentations. Glycemic control is paramount in preventing diabetic peripheral neuropathy and cardiac autonomic neuropathy in T1DM. Glycemic control can slow the progression of

---

Box 15
Lipid recommendations

Screening: ADULTS

- At diagnosis
- At initial medical evaluation
- Every 5 years, or more frequently as needed

Interventions

- Lifestyle
  - First step for ALL patients
  - Weight loss if necessary
  - Reduce saturated fat, trans fat, and cholesterol
  - Increase omega 3 fatty acids, fiber, plant stanols/sterols
  - Increase physical activity
- Triglycerides (Tg)
  - ≥150 mg/dL and high-density lipoprotein (HDL) ≤40 men, ≤50 women
    - Intensify lifestyle and optimize glycemic control
  - ≥500 fasting
    - Evaluate for secondary causes
    - Treat to reduce risk of pancreatitis; fibrates
    - NO alcohol
- Medication
  - Statins: see **Table 11** recommended statin intensity
  - Consider ezetimibe
    - Recent acute coronary syndrome AND low-density lipoprotein (LDL) ≥50 on moderate-dose statin
    - Hx of ASCVD and high-intensity statin intolerant
  - Statin/Fibrate combination
    - Not proven to improve ASCVD outcomes: not generally recommended
    - Consider in men with
      - Tg ≥204 mg/dL
      - HDL ≤34 mg/dL
  - Statin/Niacin
    - No cardiovascular benefit, may increase risk for cerebrovascular accident
    - Not recommended
  - Pregnancy
    - Do not use statins
  - PCSK9
    - Adjunct therapy for those at high risk for ASCVD who
      - Need additional LDL lowering
      - Who require but are intolerant of high-dose statins

Data from American Diabetes Association. Standards of medical care in diabetes 2017. Diabetes Care 2017;40(Suppl 1):S1–135.

---

neuropathy in T2DM, but it cannot reverse any neuronal loss or damage.[5] Patients should be evaluated for non–diabetes-related causes of neuropathy, such as toxic exposure, B12 deficiency, hypothyroidism, malignancies, infections, inherited neuropathies, and vasculitis.[5] Neuropathy recommendations are detailed in **Box 20**.

Foot Care

Ulcers and amputations are serious conditions that can disproportionately affect people with diabetes. Early diagnosis and treatment can prevent or delay serious morbidity and mortality. Recommendations for foot care are outlined in **Box 21**.

Table 11
American Diabetes Association–recommended statin intensity

ASCVD Risks	Age <40	Age 40–75	Age >75
None	None	Moderate	Moderate
ASCVD risk(s)	Moderate or high	High	Moderate or high
ASCVD	High	High	High
ACS and LDL ≥50 OR Hx ASCVD and high-dose statin intolerant		Moderate + ezetimibe	Moderate + ezetimibe

ASCVD risk factors: LDL ≥100, albuminuria, family history premature ASCVD, hypertension, smoking, chronic kidney disease.

Abbreviations: ACS, acute coronary syndrome; ASCVD, atherosclerotic cardiovascular disease; Hx, history; LDL, low-density lipoprotein.

Data from American Diabetes Association. Standards of medical care in diabetes 2017. Diabetes Care 2017;40(Suppl 1):S1–135.

OLDER ADULTS

More than 25% of the population older than 65 has diabetes.[1] It is therefore critical that health care providers are aware of the unique issues that pertain to this population.

Neurocognitive Function

Adults with diabetes who are older than 65 are at increased risk for cognitive decline and should therefore be screened annually for mild cognitive impairment and

Box 16
Aspirin recommendations

- History of ASCVD
  - 75 to 162 mg
  - If allergic, use clopidogrel 75 mg/d
- Increased risk for CVD without increased risk for bleeding
  - Consider aspirin 75 to 162 mg/d
  - Older than 50 years and 1 major risk:
    - Family Hx premature ASCVD
    - Hypertension
    - Dyslipidemia
    - Smoking
    - Albuminuria
- Younger than 50 years and no increased risk for CVD
  - ASA is NOT recommended
- Younger than 50 years AND multiple ASCVD risks
  - ASA recommended based on clinical judgment
- Younger than 21 years
  - Contraindicated due to risk of Reye syndrome
- Dual therapy
  - One year or more after acute coronary syndrome

Data from American Diabetes Association. Standards of medical care in diabetes 2017. Diabetes Care 2017;40(Suppl 1):S1–135.

Box 17
Coronary heart disease recommendations

- Screening
  - Asymptomatic persons
    - Not recommended
  - Consider in
    - Unexplained dyspnea, chest pain
    - Carotid bruits
    - Transient ischemic attack
    - Cerebrovascular accident
    - Claudication
    - Peripheral artery disease (PAD)
    - Electrocardiogram abnormalities, ie, Q waves
- Treatment
  - Known ASCVD
    - ASA and statin
    - Consider ACEI
  - Prior myocardial infarction
    - Beta blockers 2 years after event
  - Symptomatic heart failure
    - Avoid TZD
  - Stable congestive heart failure
    - Metformin OK if eGFR greater than 30
    - Avoid if unstable or while hospitalized

Data from American Diabetes Association. Standards of medical care in diabetes 2017. Diabetes Care 2017;40(Suppl 1):S1–135.

---

dementia as well as depression.[5] Drug regimens may need to be simplified and patients may need to enlist additional help with self-care tasks.

Hypoglycemia

Older patients are at increased risk for hypoglycemia due to cognitive deficits, longer duration of disease, and progressive renal insufficiency.[5] It is imperative to prevent hypoglycemia to reduce the risk of severe injury and potential further cognitive decline. Patients should be regularly assessed for hypoglycemia and medication regimens, and glucose targets need to be adjusted to avoid persistent hypoglycemia.

Treatment Goals

The care of older adults with diabetes should be tailored to their health status. Goals for A1C, glucose targets, lipids, and BP should all be individualized based on the functional status of the individual patient. Treatment goals for the older adult are detailed in the ADA standards of medical care in diabetes 2017,[5] available at: https://professional.diabetes.org/sites/professional.diabetes.org/files/media/abridged_standards_of_medical_care_in_diabetes_2017_0.pdf.

Medication use in older adults requires special consideration with regard to polypharmacy, patient preference, and cost. Some medication issues to consider by class in the elderly are listed in **Box 22**.

CHILDREN AND ADOLESCENTS

Nearly 75% of cases of T1DM are diagnosed in children and adolescents younger than 18.[5] Children and adolescents pose unique management challenges, such as variable

---

Box 18
Diabetic kidney disease (DKD) recommendations

- Screening
  - Urinary albumin-to-creatinine ratio (UACR)
    - Normal value <30
    - Spot UACR preferred
    - 24-hour collection not necessary
    - 2 of 3 specimens over 3 to 6 months need to be abnormal to diagnose albuminuria
    - Can be elevated independent of kidney damage by
      - Exercise
      - Infection
      - Fever
      - CHF
      - Marked hyperglycemia
      - Marked hypertension
      - Menstruation
  - eGFR
    - Normal greater than 60

- T1DM
  - Screen ≥5 years' duration of disease

- T2DM
  - Screen all patients

- Comorbid hypertension
  - Screen all patients

- Treatment
  - Glycemic control
  - Blood pressure control
  - DKD not on dialysis
    - Protein intake 0.8 g/kg per day
  - Comorbid hypertension (nonpregnant) and
    - ACE or ARB
      - UACR 30 to 299
        - Recommended
      - UACR >300 and/or eGFR <60
        - Strongly recommended
      - Not recommended for patients
        - Without hypertension
        - Normal UACR less than 30
        - Normal eGFR

- Monitoring
  - If using ACEI, ARB, or diuretics
    - Monitor for elevated creatinine, potassium
  - If eGFR less than 60
    - Evaluate for complications of chronic kidney disease
  - If eGFR less than 30
    - Refer for renal replacement treatment

Data from American Diabetes Association. Standards of medical care in diabetes 2017. Diabetes Care 2017;40(Suppl 1):S1–135.

---

insulin sensitivity related to growth and sexual maturation, variable capabilities for self-care, issues with child care and school environment, and vulnerability to hyperglycemia and hypoglycemia due to the reduced communication skills in the very young. Because of their unique developmental challenges, it is imperative that children,

---

Box 19
Diabetic retinopathy (DR) recommendations

Screening

- T1DM
  - Initial dilated eye examination within 5 years after diagnosis
- T2DM
  - Initial dilated eye examination at diagnosis
- Retinopathy
  - Not present for 1 + examination and good glycemic control
    - Dilated examination every 2 years
  - If present
    - Dilated examination every year
  - If worsening or sight-threatening
    - More frequently per ophthalmology
- Pregnancy in preexisting T1DM and T2DM
  - Risk for development or progression of DR
  - Dilated eye examination before conception or in first trimester
  - Monitored every trimester
  - Monitored for 1 year postpartum as necessitated by the degree of DR

Treatment

- Refer to experienced ophthalmologist for any
  - Macular edema
  - Severe nonproliferative DR
  - Proliferative DR
- Laser photocoagulation indicated for
  - Severe nonproliferative DR
  - Proliferative DR
- Intravitreal injections
  - Antivascular endothelial growth factor for central-involved macular edema
- Aspirin therapy for cardio protection
  - NOT contraindicated in DR
  - Does not increase risk of retinal hemorrhage

Data from American Diabetes Association. Standards of medical care in diabetes 2017. Diabetes Care 2017;40(Suppl 1):S1–135.

---

adolescents, and their caregivers are cared for by a multidisciplinary team that is familiar with both diabetes and pediatric patients.

Education
- All youth and caregivers
  - DSME and DSMS that is culturally and developmentally appropriate

Psychosocial
- Assess for psychosocial issues and family stressors
  - Refer to mental health provider as necessary
- Developmentally appropriate involvement of diabetes tasks
  - Do not transfer care over to the child until the child is ready
- Referral to mental health for
  - Behavioral self-care difficulties

Box 20
Neuropathy recommendations

Screening for diabetic peripheral neuropathy

- T1DM
  - 5 years after diagnosis
  - Then annually
- T2DM
  - At diagnosis
  - Then annually

Diagnosis

- Assessment for distal symmetric polyneuropathy should include
  - Small fiber function
    - Produce most common early symptoms
      - Pain
      - Dysthesias
        - Burning
        - Tingling
    - Evaluate
      - Temperature
      - Pinprick sensation
  - Large fiber function
    - Produce later symptoms
      - Numbness
      - Loss of protective sensation
        - Risk for ulcer
    - Vibration sense with 128-Hz
  - 10-g monofilament
    - Annual to identify at-risk feet

- Diabetic autonomic neuropathy
  - Assess for in patients with microvascular and neuropathic complications
  - Symptoms include
    - Hypoglycemia unawareness
    - Resting tachycardia
    - Orthostatic hypotension
    - Gastroparesis
    - Constipation
    - Erectile dysfunction
    - Neurogenic bladder
    - Sudomotor dysfunction with increased or decreased sweating

Treatment

- Glycemic control
- Neuropathic pain
  - Pregabalin
  - Duloxetine

Data from American Diabetes Association. Standards of medical care in diabetes 2017. Diabetes Care 2017;40(Suppl 1):S1–135.

  - Repeated hospitalizations for DKA
  - Eating disorders
- Adolescents age 12
  - Begin to have solo interactions with provider
- Girls at puberty
  - Begin preconception counseling

Box 21
Foot-care recommendations

Screening

- Comprehensive evaluation annually
  - Identify risks for ulcers/amputations
    - Poor glycemic control
    - Peripheral neuropathy with loss of protective sensation
    - Cigarette use
    - Foot deformities
    - Callus or corn
    - PAD
    - History of ulcer
    - Amputation
    - Visual impairment
    - Nephropathy, particularly on dialysis

Examination

- Inspect skin

- Assess for deformities

- Neurologic examination
  - Monofilament
    - Most useful to detect loss of protective sensation
  - + 1 additional
    - Pinprick
    - Temperature
    - Vibration
    - Ankle reflexes

- Vascular examination
  - Pedal pulses

- Education
  - Inspect feet daily

- Refer to specialist
  - Older than 50 + claudication, diminished pulses
  - Specialized footwear
    - Sever neuropathy
    - Foot deformities
    - Amputations

Treatment

- Proper-fitting shoes

- Molded shoes
  - Only for those with deformity

Data from American Diabetes Association. Standards of medical care in diabetes 2017. Diabetes Care 2017;40(Suppl 1):S1–135.

Glycemic Targets

The glycemic recommendations for children and adolescents (**Table 12**) reflect their increased vulnerability to hypoglycemia with less stringent glycemic targets.

Autoimmune Conditions

Persons with T1DM are at increased risk for certain other autoimmune disorders. Screening for those disorders is recommended as follows:

Box 22
DM medication issues by class in the elderly

Metformin

- First-line agent
- Ok for eGFR $\geq$30
- Contraindicated in
  - Advanced renal insufficiency
  - Heart failure
- Temporary hold for
  - Contrast procedures
  - Hospitalization
  - Acute illness

Thiazolidinediones (TZDs)

- Limited use in elderly
- Risk for edema and fractures
- Caution in
  - CHF
  - Fall risk

Insulin Secretagogues

- Risk for hypoglycemia
- Use drugs with shorter half-life
  - Glipizide
- Avoid drugs with longer half-life
  - Glyburide
- Dose adjust for
  - Renal impairment
  - Hypoglycemia

Incretin therapies

- Dipeptidyl peptidase 4
  - Few side effects
  - Minimal hypoglycemia
  - Expensive
- GLP-1 agonist
  - Injection requires visual and motor skills
  - Nausea, vomiting, and weight loss
    - May not be appropriate in undernourished

Sodium-Glucose Cotransporter 2 Inhibitors

- Oral administration
- Risk for dehydration, hypotension
- Risk for infections; genital mycotic and urinary tract
- New warnings regarding DKA and amputation

Insulin

- Requires good visual and motor skills
- Risk for hypoglycemia
- May need to simplify multiple-dose regimen for cognitive decline

Data from American Diabetes Association. Standards of medical care in diabetes 2017. Diabetes Care 2017;40(Suppl 1):S1–135.

Table 12
Glycemic targets in children and adolescents with type 1 diabetes mellitus

Fasting/Preprandial	Overnight/Bedtime	A1C	Postprandial
90–130 mg/dL	90–150 mg/dL	<7.5% <7.0% if possible without hypoglycemia	Check if discrepancy between AC glucose and A1C

Data from American Diabetes Association. Standards of medical care in diabetes 2017. Diabetes Care 2017;40(Suppl 1):S1–135.

Thyroid
- Soon after diagnosis evaluate
  - Thyroid antibodies
  - Thyroid-stimulating hormone
    - Once normoglycemic
    - If normal, repeat yearly

Celiac
- Soon after diagnosis evaluate
  - Tissue transglutaminase or gliadin
  - Immunoglobulin A
- Biopsy-confirmed celiac
  - Gluten-free diet

As for adults with diabetes, children and adolescents require assessment and management of CV risk factors. Recommendations for HTN and hyperlipidemia in children and adolescents are found in **Boxes 23** and **24**.

Tobacco use
- Assess for use at every visit
- Discourage use
- Encourage cessation

Children and adolescents with T1DM are also at risk for the development of microvascular complications. It is well documented that intensive glycemic control can prevent and delay the development of these complications.[18] Screening for microvascular complications is recommended as follows:

Nephropathy
- Screening
  - Annual for albuminuria
    - Beginning 5 years after diagnosis
  - eGFR
    - Initial evaluation
- Treatment
  - Urinary albumin-to-creatinine ratio (UACR) greater than 30 on 2 of 3 samples
    - Angiotensin-converting enzyme inhibitor
    - Glucose control

Retinopathy
- Screening
  - Comprehensive dilated eye examination
    - Initial examination

Box 23
Hypertension recommendations in children and adolescents

- Screening
  - Monitor blood pressure each visit
  - High normal
    - ≥90th percentile
  - Hypertension
    - ≥ 95th percentile
  - Confirm reading on 3 separate days

- Treatment
  - High normal ≥90th percentile
    - Dietary modification
      - Weight control if applicable
    - Exercise
    - 3-month trial
      - If not improved, pharmacology
  - High normal ≥95th percentile
    - Lifestyle interventions
    - Pharmacology as soon as HTN confirmed
  - Medications
    - ACEI and ARB
      - First line
      - Reproductive counseling and birth control due to teratogenic effects

- Goal
  - Less than 90th percentile

Data from American Diabetes Association. Standards of medical care in diabetes 2017. Diabetes Care 2017;40(Suppl 1):S1–135.

Box 24
Hyperlipidemia recommendations in children and adolescents

- Screening
  - Older than 10 years
    - Soon after diagnosis
  - LDL greater than 100
    - Annual monitoring
  - LDL less than 100
    - Monitor ever 3 to 5 years

- Treatment
  - Glucose control
  - Medical nutrition therapy
    - Step 2 American Heart Association diet
  - Statin therapy suggested for
    - Older than 10 years
      - LDL greater than 160
      - LDL greater than 130 AND one or more cardiovascular risk factor

- Goal
  - LDL less than 100

Data from American Diabetes Association. Standards of medical care in diabetes 2017. Diabetes Care 2017;40(Suppl 1):S1–135.

- After having diabetes 3 to 5 years, once the child is 10 years or older or puberty has started, whichever is first
  - Annual examination thereafter
    - May reduce on recommendation of ophthalmology

Neuropathy
- Foot examination
  - Annual examination
    - After having diabetes for 5 years and is 10 years or older or puberty has started, whichever is first

TYPE 2 DIABETES IN YOUTH

T2DM was previously a disease almost exclusively in adults; however, over the past 20 years, the incidence of T2DM has been rapidly increasing in youth. T2DM in youth differs from the disease in adults in that there is typically more rapid beta cell decline and more rapid development of complications in the younger population.[5]

Diagnostic criteria for T2DM are the same as for adults (see **Table 4**). Treatment goals are the same for youth with T1DM and T2DM (see **Table 12**). Medication options for youth with T2DM are limited to insulin and metformin. Unlike T1DM, which typically has a rapid onset, T2DM can take years to develop. Children with T2DM may therefore already have complications of the disease upon diagnosis. The following data should be obtained at the initial visit:

- BP measurement
- Fasting lipid profile
- Spot UACR
- Dilated eye examination

PREGNANCY

Please see previous section (Diagnosis: Gestational Diabetes) for the guidelines on the diagnosis of GDM.

In women without diabetes, pregnancy alters normal glucose metabolism. Fasting glucose levels are lower than the nonpregnant state due to insulin-independent glucose use by the fetus and placenta as well as by postprandial hyperglycemia and carbohydrate intolerance resulting from placental hormones.[5] Women with GDM are at greater risk for macrosomia, birth complications, and persistent diabetes after pregnancy.

Recommendations for the care of the pregnant woman with preexisting T1DM and T2DM are found in **Box 25**.

Recommendations for the care of the pregnant woman with GDM are found in **Box 26**.

General recommendations for the care of the pregnant woman with GDM are found in **Box 27**.

GLYCEMIC TARGETS IN GESTATIONAL DIABETES AND PREEXISTING TYPE 1 DIABETES OR TYPE 2 DIABETES IN PREGNANCY

The ADA recommends unified glycemic targets for pregnant women regardless if they have GDM, T1DM, or T2DM.[5] **Table 13** outlines the ADA glycemic targets for GDM, T1DM, and T2DM.

Box 25
Recommendations for the care of the pregnant woman with preexisting T1DM and T2DM

- Preconception counseling
  - Beginning at puberty for all girls
  - Emphasize importance of glycemic control
    - A1C <6.5%
  - Discuss risk for development/progression of DR
    - Dilated eye examination
      - Before conception or during first trimester
      - Monitor each trimester
      - Continue 1 year post delivery
  - Medications
    - Insulin
      - Preferred
  - Hypoglycemia
    - T1DM
      - Increased risk during pregnancy due to altered counterregulatory response

Data from American Diabetes Association. Standards of medical care in diabetes 2017. Diabetes Care 2017;40(Suppl 1):S1–135.

Unlike the ADA, AACE differentiates glycemic targets between GDM and preexisting T1DM and T2DM.[25] **Table 14** provides the AACE glycemic targets in pregnancy.

DIABETES CARE IN THE HOSPITAL

Hyperglycemia in the hospital setting is defined as glucose levels consistently greater than 140 mg/dL.[5] Hospitalized patients who experience hypoglycemia and hyperglycemia are at significant risk for serious adverse events, including infections, arrhythmias, and even death.[5] It is therefore imperative that glycemia is managed appropriately in the hospital setting. Treatment should be initiated for glucose values persistently greater than 180. Insulin is the preferred treatment for hyperglycemia in hospitalized patients. Sliding scale insulin as the sole treatment for hyperglycemia is strongly discouraged. Recommendations for diabetes care in the hospital are found in **Box 28**.

Box 26
Recommendations for the care of the pregnant woman with gestational diabetes (GDM)

Gestational diabetes

- Lifestyle change is foundation
  - Potentially 70% to 80% controlled with lifestyle alone

- Medication
  - Insulin is preferred treatment
  - Metformin and glyburide may be used but do cross placenta

- Follow-up
  - Repeat oral glucose tolerance test 4 to 12 weeks postpartum
    - If normal, repeat diabetes screening every 1 to 3 years
  - High risk to develop T2DM
  - Metformin and lifestyle interventions shown to prevent or delay progression to DM

Data from American Diabetes Association. Standards of medical care in diabetes 2017. Diabetes Care 2017;40(Suppl 1):S1–135.

Box 27
General recommendations for the care of the pregnant woman with GDM

- Medications to avoid in childbearing women not using reliable contraception
  - ACEI, statin
- Glucose monitoring
  - Fasting and postprandial
    - GDM and preexisting
  - Preprandial monitoring
    - Preexisting DM
- A1C
  - Lower in pregnant than nonpregnant women due to high red blood cell turnover
  - Goal 6.0% to 6.5%
  - Less than 6%
    - Optimal if achieved without hypoglycemia
- Blood pressure
  - With chronic hypertension
    - Goal 120 to 160/80 to 105
    - Avoid ACEI

Data from American Diabetes Association. Standards of medical care in diabetes 2017. Diabetes Care 2017;40(Suppl 1):S1–135.

Table 13
American Diabetes Association glycemic targets for gestational diabetes, type 1 diabetes, and type 2 diabetes

Fasting	One-hour Postprandial	Two-hour Postprandial	A1C
≤95 mg/dL	≤140 mg/dL	≤120 mg/dL	6.0%–6.5% <6.0% if achieved without hypoglycemia

Data from American Diabetes Association. Standards of medical care in diabetes 2017. Diabetes Care 2017;40(Suppl 1):S1–135.

Table 14
American Association of Clinical Endocrinology glycemic targets in pregnancy

	Preprandial	Postprandial	A1C
GDM	≤95 mg/dL	1-h: ≤140 mg/dL 2-h: ≤120 mg/dL	≤6.0%
Preexisting T1DM or T2DM	60–99 mg/dL Includes HS/overnight	100–129 mg/dL Peak postprandial	≤6.0%

Abbreviations: GDM, gestational diabetes; T1DM, type 1 diabetes mellitus; T2DM, type 2 diabetes mellitus.
Data from AACE Management of pregnancy complicated by diabetes. Available at: http://outpatient.aace.com/diabetes-in-pregnancy/pregnancydm-s3-management. Accessed June 1, 2017.

Box 28
Diabetes care in the hospital

- Testing
  - A1C
    - All patients with diabetes or hyperglycemia if not performed in previous 3 months
    - ≥6.5% indicates diabetes before admission
  - Bedside monitoring
    - Eating meals
      - Before meals and bedtime
    - Nothing by mouth or enteral feeding
      - Every 4 to 6 hours
    - Intravenous insulin
      - Every 30 minutes to 2 hours
  - Continuous glucose monitoring
    - Not recommended in hospital

- Glycemic targets
  - 140 to 180
    - Most hospitalized patients
  - Less than 140
    - Some stable patients, only if can achieve without hypoglycemia
  - Greater than 180
    - Older, terminally ill

- Treatment
  - Insulin therapy
    - Initiate for glucose persistently greater than 180
      - Intravenous insulin
        - Critically ill patients
        - Use validated protocols
        - Discontinue 1 to 2 hours after basal insulin administered
  - Basal insulin or basal + correction
    - Poor/unpredictable oral intake or enteral feeding
  - Basal, bolus, correctional
    - Predictable oral intake
  - Sliding scale and premixed
    - Not recommended

- Oral hypoglycemic
  - DC on admission
  - Consider resumption 1 to 2 days before DC when stable

- Hypoglycemia
  - Less than 70
    - Review treatment and adjust as necessary
  - Less than 54
    - Clinically significant hypoglycemia
  - Severe hypoglycemia
    - Any value in which patient is cognitively impaired
  - Causes
    - Reduced oral intake, emesis
    - Reduced dose of glucocorticoids
    - Decreased intravenous dextrose
    - Disruption on oral, enteral, or parenteral feeding

- Perioperative care
  - Glucose target 80 to 180 mg/dL
  - Oral agents
    - Metformin
      - Hold 24 hours preoperatively
    - Other agents
      - Hold day of

- ○ Insulin
  - ■ NPH
    - • 50% dose in morning
  - ■ Long-acting analog or pump
    - • 60% to 80% dose in morning
- • Monitoring
  - ○ Every 4 to 6 hours while NPO (nothing by mouth) and correct hyperglycemia as needed

Data from American Diabetes Association. Standards of medical care in diabetes 2017. Diabetes Care 2017;40(Suppl 1):S1–135.

Box 29
Components of diabetes discharge education

- • Arrange for follow-up care with DM provider
- • Understanding the diagnosis of diabetes/hyperglycemia, glucose monitoring, glucose targets, when to call provider
- • Recognizing the signs, symptoms, and treatment of hypoglycemia
- • Recognizing the signs, symptoms, and treatment of hyperglycemia
- • Nutrition guidance
- • Medication reconciliation
- • Medication instruction
- • Sick day management
- • Proper use of equipment, such as glucometer, needles, and disposal

Data from American Diabetes Association. Standards of medical care in diabetes 2017. Diabetes Care 2017;40(Suppl 1):S1–135.

The transition from hospital to home can be very stressful for patients and caregivers. Before discharge, patients need to receive diabetes-focused education.[5] See **Box 29** for the minimal components of diabetes discharge education.

SUMMARY

Diabetes is a complicated group of disorders that requires knowledgeable providers and engaged patients to collaborate within a patient-centered team approach for optimal outcomes.

This article is intended to guide practice but does not substitute for clinical judgment. These recommendations should be considered within the context of individual patient preferences, comorbidities, and prognoses and adapted as necessary to develop a specific plan of care that is customized for each patient.

REFERENCES

1. Centers for Disease Control and Prevention. 2014 National Diabetes Statistics Report. Available at: https://www.cdc.gov/diabetes/data/statistics/2014statistics-report.html. Accessed January 13, 2017.

2. Centers for Disease Control and Prevention. National Center for Health Statistics. Age differences in visits to office-based physicians by patients with diabetes:

United States, 2010. Available at: https://www.cdc.gov/nchs/data/databriefs/db161.htm. Accessed February 3, 2017.

3. Centers for Disease Control and Prevention. Diabetes Public Health Resource. Distribution of first-listed diagnoses among hospital discharges with diabetes as any-listed diagnosis, adults aged 18 years and older, United States, 2010. Available at: https://www.cdc.gov/diabetes/statistics/hosp/adulttable1.htm. Accessed February 8, 2017.

4. Young-Hymann D, de Groot M, Hill-Briggs F, et al. Psychosocial care for people with diabetes: a position statement of the American Diabetes Association. Diabetes Care 2016;39(12):2126–40.

5. American Diabetes Association. Standards of medical care in diabetes 2017. Diabetes Care 2017;40(Suppl 1):S1–135.

6. Zhang X, Gregg EW, Williamson DF, et al. A1C level and future risk of diabetes: a systematic review. Diabetes Care 2010;33:1665–73.

7. American Association of Clinical Endocrinologists. Diagnosis of type 2 diabetes mellitus. Available at: http://outpatient.aace.com/type-2-diabetes/diagnosis-of-type2-diabetes-mellitus. Accessed May 1, 2017.

8. Expert Committee on the Diagnosis and Classification of Diabetes Mellitus. Report of the Expert Committee on the Diagnosis and Classification of Diabetes Mellitus. Diabetes Care 1997;20:1183–97.

9. Suh S, Kim K-W. Diabetes and cancer: is diabetes causally related to cancer? Diabetes Metab J 2011;35:193–8.

10. Smith KJ, Beland M, Clyde M, et al. Association of diabetes with anxiety: a systematic review and meta-analysis. J Psychosom Res 2013;74:89–99.

11. Anderson RJ, Freedland KE, Clouse RE, et al. The prevalence of comorbid depression in adults with diabetes: a meta-analysis. Diabetes Care 2001;24:1069–78.

12. Haas L, Maryniuk M, Beck J, et al. National standards for diabetes self-management education and support. Diabetes Care 2012;35(11):2393–401.

13. Norris SL, Lau J, Smith SJ, et al. Self-management education for adults with type 2 diabetes: a meta-analysis of the effect on glycemic control. Diabetes Care 2002;25:1159–71.

14. Balk EM, Earley A, Raman G, et al. Combined diet and physical activity promotion programs to prevent type 2 diabetes among persons at increased risk: a systematic review for the Community Preventive Services Task Force. Ann Intern Med 2015;164:164–75.

15. Stanton CA, Keith DR, Gaalema DE, et al. Trends in tobacco use among US adults with chronic health conditions: National Survey on Drug Use and Health 2005-2013. Prev Med 2016;92:160–8.

16. Aikens JE. Prospective associations between emotional distress and poor outcomes in type 2 diabetes. Diabetes Care 2012;35:2472–8.

17. Lindström J, Ilanne-Parikka P, Peltonen M, et al, Finnish Diabetes Prevention Study Group. Sustained reduction in the incidence of type 2 diabetes by lifestyle intervention: follow-up of the Finnish Diabetes Prevention Study. Lancet 2006;368:1673–9.

18. The Diabetes Control and Complications Trial Research Group. The effect of intensive treatment of diabetes on the development and progression of long-term complications in insulin-dependent diabetes mellitus. N Engl J Med 1993;329:977–86.

19. UK Prospective Diabetes Study (UKPDS) Group. Intensive blood-glucose control with sulphonylureas or insulin compared with conventional treatment and risk of

complications in patients with type 2 diabetes (UKPDS 33). Lancet 1998;352: 837–53.

20. Knowler WC, Barrett-Connor E, Fowler SE, et al, Diabetes Prevention Program Research Group. Reduction in the incidence of type 2 diabetes with lifestyle intervention or metformin. N Engl J Med 2002;346:393–403.
21. Goldstein DJ. Beneficial health effects of modest weight loss. Int J Obes Relat Metab Disord 1992;16:397–415.
22. Rubino F, Nathan DM, Eckel RH, et al, Delegates of the 2nd Diabetes Surgery Summit. Metabolic surgery in the treatment algorithm for type 2 diabetes: a joint statement by international diabetes organizations. Diabetes Care 2016;39: 861–77.
23. Garber AJ, Abrahamson MJ, Barzilay JI, et al. Consensus statement by the American Association of Clinical Endocrinologists and American College of Endocrinology on the comprehensive type 2 diabetes management algorithm—2017 executive summary. Endocr Pract 2017;23(2):207–38.
24. Tuttle KR, Bakris GL, Bilous RW, et al. Diabetic kidney disease: a report from an ADA Consensus Conference. Diabetes Care 2014;37:2864–83.
25. AACE Management of pregnancy complicated by diabetes. Available at: http:// outpatient.aace.com/diabetes-in-pregnancy/pregnancydm-s3-management. Accessed June 1, 2017.

Prediabetes
Beyond the Borderline

Mara Lynn Wilson, RN, MS, FNP-C, CDE

KEYWORDS

- Prediabetes • Impaired fasting glucose (IFG) • Impaired glucose tolerance (IGT)

KEY POINTS

- Prediabetes is a complex multifactorial metabolic disorder that extends beyond glucose control.
- Prediabetes is not the harmless condition that it was previously thought to be.
- Microvascular and microvascular changes are present with the onset of glycemic dysregulation.
- Identification and intervention can reverse or delay the progression of prediabetes.

INTRODUCTION

Defined by the American Diabetes Association (ADA) in 1997, prediabetes recognizes those specific individuals who did not meet the diagnostic criteria of type 2 diabetes (T2DM) but whose laboratory testing levels were not at normal values.[1] Prediabetes is a complex multifactorial metabolic disorder that extends beyond glucose control.[2] Once thought of as an innocuous condition, current studies have found that microvascular (neuropathy, nephropathy, and retinopathy), macrovascular (stroke, coronary artery disease, and peripheral vascular disease), periodontal disease, cognitive dysfunction, blood pressure changes, obstructive sleep apnea, low testosterone level, fatty liver disease, and cancer are some of conditions that are present with the onset of glycemic dysregulation.[3–5] The presence of prediabetes increases the risk of developing T2DM by 3-fold to 10-fold.[3] Worldwide it is estimated that 5% to 10% of people with prediabetes will develop T2DM, whereas an American Diabetes Association expert panel estimates up to 70% will progress to T2DM.[4] Once the diagnosis of T2DM is made the condition cannot be reversed or cured but it can be controlled.[6]

Disclosure: The author has nothing to disclose.
Department of Endocrine Neoplasia and Hormonal Disorder, MD Anderson Cancer Center, 1400 Pressler Street, Room FCT 12.5039.02, Houston, TX 77030-3722, USA
E-mail address: MLWilson1@MDAnderson.org

DIAGNOSIS

Prediabetes is diagnosed using the following criteria (**Box 1**):

- Impaired fasting glucose (IFG) as defined by a fasting glucose level between 100 mg/dL and 125 mg/dL
- Impaired glucose tolerance (IGT) as defined by a glucose level between 140 and 199 mg/dL 2-hours after receiving a 75-g oral glucose tolerance test (OGTT)
- Hemoglobin A1c 5.7% to 6.4%

The A1c is a simple test to obtain; many clinics and offices have the ability to obtain results in less than 15 minutes with point-of-care (POC) technology. The ADA does not recommend the POC A1c for diagnostic purpose at this time because there is no current proficiency testing mandate for performing the test.[1] It is important to obtain an accurate medical history because the hemoglobin A1c results can be inaccurate in the presence of certain conditions. Conditions such as asplenia, iron deficiency anemia, vitamin B_{12} and folate deficiency anemias can falsely increase the A1c results.[7] In contrast, hemoglobin A1c results can be falsely decreased in the following conditions: pregnancy, acute and chronic blood loss, hemolytic anemia, splenomegaly, and end-stage renal failure.[7] If a patient has one of these conditions the diagnosis of prediabetes or diabetes should be made using other diagnostic criteria.

RISK FACTORS

The main risk factors for diabetes are divided into 3 categories: modifiable, unmodifiable, and other.

Unmodifiable risk factors include:

- Family history or first-degree relative with T2DM
- Ethnicity (Native American, African American, Hispanic, Asian American, and Pacific Islander)
- Age

Modifiable risk factors include:

- Being overweight or obese. Body mass index (BMI) more than 25 kg/m^2
- Physical inactivity

Other risk factors include:

- History of gestational diabetes
- Delivery of a child weighing more than 9 pounds (4.1 kg)
- Hypertension
- Dyslipidemia

Box 1
Diagnosis of prediabetes

Fasting glucose level between 100 mg/dL and 125 mg/dL, or

Two-hour post–75-g oral glucose tolerance test between 140 and 199 mg/dL, or

Hemoglobin A1c between 5.7% and 6.4%

Adapted from American Diabetes Association. Standards of medical care in diabetes–2017. The journal of Clinical and applied research and education 2017;40 (Suppl 1).

There is a 93% increase in the development of T2DM as the BMI increases from 23 to greater than 35 kg/m^2.[8]

INCIDENCE

An estimated 86 million people in the United States have prediabetes; according to the 2010 census data this number equates to the total state populations of California, Texas, New York, and Oregon combined.[1,9] The increased incidence of prediabetes is directly related to physical inactivity and the increased rates of obesity. Prediabetes increased between 2010 and 2014, from 35% in those aged more than 20 years (50% of those >65 years of age) to 37% in those more than 20 years of age (51% in those >65 years of age).[10,11] The populations with the highest risk of prediabetes included non-Hispanic black people (39.6%) non-Hispanic white people (38.2%), and Mexican Americans (38%).[12] As the United States population ages, the incidence of age-related conditions such as prediabetes and T2DM will continue to increase.[13] Prevention of prediabetes and T2DM is crucial to reverse the impending epidemic.[6,13]

ECONOMIC IMPACT

The annual direct cost in 2012 of care of a person with prediabetes was $510; undiagnosed T2DM was $4030; and diagnosed diabetes was $10,970.[6] Cost of care of individuals with T2DM is related to the increased incidence of morbidity and mortality associated with macrovascular disease and microvascular disease.[10] The direct and indirect (reduced quality of life, reduced employment, absenteeism, and decreased productivity)[3,6] health care expenses in 2012 were in excess of $245 billion.[10] Prediabetes and diabetes and their complications will continue to cause an increase in total health care expenditures if current trends are not slowed or reversed, and the socioeconomic implications are alarming. Only prevention can mitigate the cost of care and increase the quality of life for the US population.[13]

NORMAL METABOLISM

In people without prediabetes or diabetes, glucose control is highly regulated by multiple hormones, including glucagon (secreted from pancreatic α cells) and insulin (secreted from pancreatic beta cells). The presence of glucose stimulates insulin production, which then inhibits production of glucagon and thus decreases hepatic output of glucose. The secretion of insulin is biphasic and is classified as first and second phase. The first-phase insulin response is activated as a direct response to a meal and consists of a spike that last approximately 10 minutes.[14] The first phase is closely followed by the second phase, in which there is a gradual secretion of insulin that reaches steady state after 1 to 2 hours depending on the degree of hyperglycemia.[14] The principal site of postprandial glucose uptake is the skeletal muscle.[15] In simplest terms, the insulin then "unlocks the door to the cell," allowing glucose to enter and provide energy (**Fig. 1**).

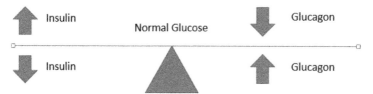

Fig. 1. Normal glucose control.

ERRORS IN METABOLISM

Prediabetes is associated with increased glucose levels, decreased beta-cell function, and decreased insulin resistance.[2] Insulin resistance is defined as a condition in which the normal insulin concentration does not adequately produce a normal insulin response in the peripheral target tissues, such as adipose tissues, muscle, and liver.[2,16] This lack of response leads to decreased uptake of glucose in those tissues and increases circulating glucose levels. The resulting hyperglycemia causes the beta cells in the pancreas to secrete more insulin to overcome the resistance. Initially the beta cells are able to maintain euglycemia. Over time, the beta-cell function diminishes and the glucose level begins to increase. The increased glucose level is first manifested as an increase in the postprandial glucose level followed by changes in the fasting glucose level.[2]

Insulin resistance in the liver leads to an overproduction of hepatic glucose output, which is stimulated through the process of gluconeogenesis. The pancreatic α cells continue to produce glucagon in spite of increased circulating insulin levels. Severe hepatic insulin resistance is present when there is an increase in glucose output despite a 2-fold to 3-fold increase of insulin production.[2]

IMPAIRED GLUCOSE TOLERANCE

Individuals with IGT have decreased first-phase and second-phase insulin responses during OGTT.[5,17] The OGTT is performed after an overnight fast. A fasting glucose level is obtained and then a 75-g glucose solution is consumed. The glucose levels are collected at 1 hour, 2 hours, and 3 hours. The OGTT is able to assess the degree of dysfunction of the beta cells under real-life conditions.[18] Some people with IGT have lost greater than 80% of their beta-cell function.[2] The site of resistance is the muscle, with small changes noted in the liver.[4,5]

IMPAIRED FASTING GLUCOSE

Fasting glucose samples are easily obtained. However, fasting glucose levels do not provide insight into the degree of dysfunction of the beta cells.[18] Studies have found that individuals with IFG have impaired early insulin responses (decreased first phase) during OGTT, which improve during the second phase of the test.[5,17] The site of resistance is the liver, with small changes in the muscle cells.[5,17]

The presence of both IGT and IFG increases the risk of developing T2DM.[5] People with the highest A1c levels were more likely to progress from prediabetes to T2DM over 5 years.[19] The presence of increased A1c level in addition to IFG or IGT also increased the risk of progression.[19]

INSULIN RESISTANCE–RELATED DISORDERS

IFG levels and IGT have also been associated with other conditions, such as polycystic ovarian syndrome, gestational diabetes, and metabolic syndrome.

POLYCYSTIC OVARIAN SYNDROME

Polycystic ovarian syndrome is associated with insulin resistance, infertility, obesity, dyslipidemia, and hypertension, and is diagnosed in approximately 5% of women of childbearing age.[20] Diagnosis of polycystic ovarian syndrome increases the risk of being diagnosed with gestational diabetes and T2DM.[1,3]

GESTATIONAL DIABETES

The increased rate of obesity has been directly related to increased incidence of gestational diabetes.[1] Gestational diabetes has been associated with both maternal and fetal risk.[1] Maternal risk includes macrosomia, increased rates of preeclampsia, and cesarean section.[1] Neonatal risk includes hypoglycemia and hyperbilirubinemia.[1] The effects of gestational diabetes linger after delivery. Up to 70% of women who were diagnosed with gestational diabetes progressed to T2DM.[21,22] There may be an increased risk of obesity and T2DM in infants born to mothers who were diagnosed with gestational diabetes.[1]

METABOLIC SYNDROME

Persons with prediabetes often have corresponding risk factors associated with metabolic syndrome. These risk factors include IGT, central obesity, high triglyceride levels, low levels of high-density lipoprotein (HDL), and hypertension (**Table 1**). Approximately 50% of patients with prediabetes meet criteria for the diagnosis of metabolic syndrome, which increases the risk of developing T2DM 5-fold.[3,16] Metabolic syndrome seems to be the link between prediabetes and macrovascular disease.[14]

SCREENING/TESTING GUIDELINES

The ADA recommends that an informal assessment of risk factors should be considered in asymptomatic adults.[1] The US Centers for Disease Control and Prevention (CDC) have developed a 7-question screening test that is simple to administer and

Table 1 International Diabetes Federation metabolic syndrome worldwide definition	
Clinical Findings	
Central obesity	BMI>30 kg/m^2 or Waist circumference: ethnicity specific European, South and Central Americas, sub-Saharan Africans, eastern Mediterranean, and Middle Eastern: Men ≥94 cm Women ≥80 cm South Asian and Chinese: Men ≥90 cm Women ≥80 cm Japanese: Men ≥85 cm Women ≥90 cm Plus any 2 of the following:
Insulin resistance	Fasting plasma >100 mg/dL; if glucose level is >100 mg/dL the OGTT is recommended but not necessary Or previously diagnosed T2DM
Blood pressure	≥130/85 mm Hg or treatment of previously diagnosed hypertension
Increased triglyceride level	≥150 mg/dL or treatment of this lipid abnormality
Reduced HDL-cholesterol	<40 mg/dL in men or <50 mg/dL in women or treatment of this lipid abnormality

Data from Alberti KGMM, Zimmet P, Shaw J. Metabolic syndrome–a new world-wide definition. A Consensus Statement from the International Diabetes Federation. Diabet Med 2006;23(5):469–80.

interpret; a score greater than 9 indicates a greater risk of developing prediabetes[23] (**Table 2**). This questionnaire is available in both English and Spanish.

The ADA and American Association of Clinical Endocrinologists (AACE) recommends testing in adults less than 45 years of age with a BMI greater than or equal to 25 kg/m² or those of Asian American descent with a BMI greater than or equal to 23 kg/m² with 1 or more risk factors[1,3]:

- A1c greater than or equal to 5.7%
- First-degree relative with diabetes
- High-risk race (eg, African American, Hispanic, Native American, Asian American, or Pacific Islander)
- History of metabolic syndrome
- History of cardiovascular disease
- Blood pressure more than 140/90 mm Hg or on therapy for hypertension
- Triglyceride level greater than or equal to 250 mg/dL or HDL less than or equal to 35 mg/dL
- Women with history of polycystic ovarian syndrome
- Personal history of gestational diabetes
- Women who have delivered a baby weighing more than 4.1 kg (9 pounds)
- Physical inactivity/sedentary lifestyle
- Persons receiving antipsychotic therapy for bipolar disease or schizophrenia
- Presence of other clinical conditions associated with insulin resistance
  - Severe obesity
  - Acanthosis nigricans

Testing is recommended in all adults more than 45 years of age. If the results are normal, testing should be repeated every 3 years.[1] In addition, testing should be considered in children and adolescents who are overweight or obese (defined as being ≥85th percentile on the growth chart) and 2 or more diabetes risk factors.[1,24] After screening/testing is completed, people should be educated on their results. A 2013 CDC report found that only 11.1% of people who met criteria for prediabetes were aware of their situation.[25]

RISK ASSOCIATED WITH PREDIABETES

Current studies have found that increased circulating levels of the inflammatory markers high-sensitivity C-reactive protein, interleukin (IL)-6, IL-18, and IL-1 receptor

Table 2
Centers for Disease Control and Prevention prediabetes screening test

Yes	No	Questions
1	0	Did you give birth to child that weighed more than 4.1 kg (9 pounds)?
1	0	Do you have a sibling (brother or sister) with T2DM?
1	0	Do you have a parent with T2DM?
5	0	Is your BMI >27 kg/m²?
5	0	Do you get little or no exercise each day and are younger than 65 y?
5	0	Is your age between 45 and 64 y?
9	0	Are you aged >65 y?

Adapted from Translation NCfCDPaHPDoD. In: Test CPS, editor: Centers for Disease Control and Prevention. Available at: https://www.cdc.gov/diabetes/prevention/pdf/prediabetestest.pdf. Accessed April 29, 2017.

antagonist (IL-1RA) were associated with higher fasting glucose levels and increased insulin resistance.[17,26] There were measurable changes in the inflammatory and immunologic markers as people progressed from euglycemia to prediabetes and then to T2DM.[26] These inflammatory changes are directly associated with the complications associated with the complications of prediabetes and T2DM.[26]

Studies have found evidence of both microvascular and macrovascular changes with the onset of glycemic dysregulation.[3,27] Microvascular changes associated with prediabetes include nephropathy leading to chronic kidney disease, neuropathy, erectile dysfunction, changes in sympathetic and parasympathetic nerve fibers, and retinopathy.[5,17,27] A recent study found that "brain changes suggestive of cerebral microvascular dysfunction are already apparent in patients with prediabetes."[28] page 1 Macrovascular changes leading to increased rates of cardiovascular disease, stroke, and peripheral vascular disease are directly associated with prediabetes.[5,10,29] Prediabetes has also been associated with periodontal disease, increased blood pressure, obstructive sleep apnea, male hypogonadism, and cancer.[5]

PREVENTION AND TREATMENT

The fundamental objective in the identification and treatment prediabetes is to:

1. Mitigate the risk associated with prediabetes and/or
2. Prevent or delay progression to T2DM[17]

T2DM was the seventh leading cause of death in 2015.[30] According to the 2014 National Diabetes Statistics Report, 9.3% or 29.1 million Americans have T2DM, which was an increase from 8.3% or 25.8 million in 2011.[10,11] If current trends continue it is projected that, by 2050, 33% of the US population will be diagnosed with T2DM.[13]

Therapeutic lifestyle modifications that target obesity, increase physical inactivity, and promote healthy eating are the foundation of the prevention and treatment of both prediabetes and diabetes.[17,31,32] The major study in the United States was the Diabetes Prevention Program (DPP), a multicenter randomized controlled trial that had 3 treatment arms (structured intensive lifestyle intervention, metformin, and placebo).[33] Lifestyle intervention decreased the development of T2DM by 58%.[33] Subsequent worldwide studies have found that therapeutic lifestyle changes have benefits that can prevent the progression from prediabetes to T2DM.[31,32,34,35] These benefits have been found to have a sustained effect for 10 to 20 years after the modifications were made.[31,34,35]

WEIGHT LOSS

Weight loss has been associated with decreased insulin resistance, decreased fasting glucose levels, and increased insulin sensitivity.[36] The weight loss needs to be maintained; as weight is regained there is a return to initial levels.[36] In persons with both prediabetes and diabetes a conservative weight loss goal of 5% to 10% should be targeted.[3,37] A minimum of 5% should be targeted because a recent meta-analysis found that weight loss of less than 5% did not improve glycemic control.[38] A decreased cardiovascular risk was found with a 7% reduction in weight in the DPP.[33]

INCREASING ACTIVITY

The World Health Organization (WHO) recommends that children and adolescents should have a minimum of 60 minutes of moderate to intense activities on a daily basis.[39] The 2017 ADA recommendations state that extended sitting should be interrupted every 30 minutes with short periods of activity.[1]

Activity for those between 18 and 64 years of age should be increased to moderate intensity for a minimum of 150 minutes a week (30 minutes on 5 days) or 75 minutes of vigorous intensity a week.[3,17,39] The same recommendation applies for adults more than 65 years of age, but muscle strengthening and balance exercise should also be added.[39]

Moderate-intensity activities include[39,40]:

- Brisk walking (5 km/h [3 miles/h]; not race walking)
- Water aerobics
- Bicycling slower than 6 km/h (10 miles/h)
- Tennis (doubles)
- Ballroom dancing
- General gardening

Vigorous intensity activities include[40]:

- Race walking, jogging, or running
- Swimming laps
- Tennis (singles)
- Aerobic dancing
- Bicycling faster than 6 km/h (10 miles/h)
- Jumping rope
- Heavy gardening (continuous digging or hoeing)
- Hiking uphill or with a heavy backpack

HEALTHY EATING

A small randomized controlled trial found that 100% of patients with prediabetes regressed to euglycemia on OGTT after following a high-protein diet (30% protein, 30% fat, and 40% carbohydrate) compared with those who followed a high-carbohydrate diet (15% protein, 30% fat, and 55% carbohydrate).[8]

A healthy diet that reduces calories and increases fiber to a minimum of 20 g should be followed.[3,39] Sources of fiber include whole-grain breads and cereals, legumes, fruits, and vegetables.[8,39] Protein sources should include lean meats, fish, chicken, egg whites, and non-fat or low-fat dairy items such as fat-free milk and low-fat cheeses.[8] The WHO recommends limiting the saturated fat to less than 10% and intake of free sugars should be less than 5% to 10% of daily caloric intake.[39] Dietary sources of fat should mainly include monounsaturated and polyunsaturated fats, including plant-based liquid oils, nuts, and fish (salmon, herring, tuna, and trout)[8]

SMOKING CESSATION

Emerging evidence is showing a link between the development of diabetes and tobacco use.[39] Smoking cessation is recommended for all persons with or without prediabetes.

MEDICATIONS

At present, there are no medications that have been approved by the US Food and Drug Administration for prediabetes.[3] A few medications that have been approved for use in T2DM have been used off label for those patients at highest risk.[3] Medications that have been studied in conjunction with therapeutic lifestyle changes have been shown to be superior to therapeutic lifestyle changes alone.[34]

A meta-analysis found that metformin reduced new-onset diabetes by 40%; the absolute risk reduction in new-onset diabetes was 6% in 1.8 years.[20,33] Metformin has also been associated with:

- Decreased fasting glucose levels
- Weight loss (BMI reduced by 5.9%)
- Improvement of lipid levels (increased HDL; decreased low-density lipoprotein and triglycerides)
- Reduced insulin resistance by 23%[20]

The 10-year follow up to the DPP showed that use of metformin delayed the onset of diabetes by 2 years compared with placebo.[41]

Liraglutide, a glucagonlike peptide 1 (GLP-1) analog, was recently studied in overweight/obese older persons with prediabetes.[42] This study found increased weight loss, decreased systolic blood pressure, decreased fasting glucose levels, decreased peripheral insulin resistance, improvement in glucose tolerance, and decreased triglyceride levels compared with placebo.[42]

In the Study to Prevent Non–insulin-dependent Diabetes Mellitus (STOP-NIDDM) trial, acarbose decreased the progression from prediabetes to diabetes by 25%.[43] Acarbose also improved glucose tolerance, improved insulin sensitivity, and reduced the risk of major cardiovascular events.[5,43]

In the ACT NOW study, pioglitazone (a known insulin sensitizer) decreased the progression to T2DM by 72% and reversed prediabetes by 42%.[44]

Orlistat, a medication that reduces fat absorption by inhibiting gastric and pancreatic lipases, was studied in conjunction with lifestyle changes. After 4 years of treatment, the incidence of progression to diabetes was 9% with placebo versus 6.2% with orlistat; this equates to a risk reduction of 37.3%.[45]

OTHER PREVENTION TREATMENT

A proof-of-concept study found that the use of continuous positive airway pressure for 8 hours a night for patients diagnosed with obstructive sleep apnea and prediabetes has been shown to improve glucose response and insulin sensitivity.[46]

RESOURCES

There are several federally funded programs designed to assist health care providers with the management and treatment of prediabetes. Two examples are the Centers for Disease Control and Prevention (CDC) and National Institute of Diabetes and Digestive and Kidney Diseases/National Diabetes Education Program.

CENTERS FOR DISEASE CONTROL AND PREVENTION DIABETES PREVENTION PROGRAM

The DPP is a yearlong lifestyle intervention program that is available in person, online, or both through CDC-recognized programs. It is currently available in all 50 states, the District of Columbia, US Virgin islands, Puerto Rico, and US-associated Pacific Islands. It is led by specially trained coaches using a research-based curriculum. More information is available at: https://www.cdc.gov/diabetes/prevention.[47]

NATIONAL INSTITUTE OF DIABETES AND DIGESTIVE AND KIDNEY DISEASES/NATIONAL DIABETES EDUCATION PROGRAM

There are free downloadable clinical practice tools and patient resources available at: https://www.niddk.nih.gov/health-information/health-communication-programs/ndep.

For health care professionals there are resources to assist in the identification and management of patients who have prediabetes. One of the items, "GAME PLAN for Preventing T2DM: A Toolkit for Health Care Professionals and Teams," has information on:

- How and why to screen for prediabetes
- Discussion points for talking to patients diagnosed with prediabetes
- Assistance with making evidence-based therapeutic lifestyle changes
- Coding and reimbursement for prediabetes screening[48]
- Patient-focused "Your Game Plan to Prevent T2DM" aids in the setting and tracking of personal goals associated with:
  - Weight loss
  - Healthy eating
  - Increasing activity
  - Talking with health care teams and getting support

The Game Plan also has advice and tips on how to meet the goals once they have been set, and is available at: https://www.niddk.nih.gov/health-information/diabetes/overview/preventing-type-2-diabetes/game-plan.[49]

Most of the resources from the National Institute of Diabetes and Digestive and Kidney Diseases/National Diabetes Education Program are multilingual and copyright free. There are additional materials that can be ordered through the NIDDK Publications Catalog, which can be accessed at: https://catalog.niddk.nih.gov/Catalog/ndep.cfm.[50]

SUMMARY

Prediabetes is not a harmless condition, as was once thought. Microvascular and macrovascular changes are present with the onset of glycemic dysregulation. It is essential to educate people who have been diagnosed with prediabetes of the associated risk. This education empowers them to institute necessary lifestyle changes to lessen their individual risks. The institution of primary prevention is crucial at this time to mitigate the future high numbers of patients who will be diagnosed with prediabetes and T2DM.

REFERENCES

1. American Diabetes Association. Standards of medical care in diabetes–2017. The journal of Clinical and applied research and education 2017;40 (Suppl 1).

2. DeFronzo RA, Eldor R, Abdul-Ghani M. Pathophysiologic approach to therapy in patients with newly diagnosed T2DM. Diabetes Care 2013;36(Supplement 2): S127–38.

3. Garber A, Handelsman Y, Einhorn D, et al. Diagnosis and management of prediabetes in the continuum of hyperglycemia—When do the risks of diabetes begin? A Consensus Statement from the American College of Endocrinology and the American Association of Clinical Endocrinologists. Endocr Pract 2008;14(7):933–46.

4. Tabák AG, Herder C, Rathmann W, et al. Prediabetes: a high-risk state for diabetes development. Lancet 2012;379(9833):2279–90.
5. Buysschaert M, Medina JL, Bergman M, et al. Prediabetes and associated disorders. Endocrine 2015;48(2):371–93.
6. Dall TM, Yang W, Halder P, et al. The economic burden of elevated blood glucose levels in 2012: diagnosed and undiagnosed diabetes, gestational diabetes mellitus, and prediabetes. Diabetes Care 2014;37(12):3172–9.
7. Radin MS. Pitfalls in hemoglobin A1c measurement: when results may be misleading. J Gen Intern Med 2014;29(2):388–94.
8. Stentz FB, Brewer A, Wan J, et al. Remission of pre-diabetes to normal glucose tolerance in obese adults with high protein versus high carbohydrate diet: randomized control trial. BMJ Open Diabetes Res Care 2016;4(1):e000258.
9. American Diabetes Association. 5. Prevention or delay of type 2 diabetes. Diabetes Care 2017;40(Supplement 1):S44–7.
10. Centers for Disease Control and Prevention. National diabetes statistics report: estimates of diabetes and its burden in the United States, 2014. Atlanta (GA): US Department of Health and Human Services; 2014.
11. Centers for Disease Control and Prevention. National diabetes fact sheet: national estimates and general information on diabetes and prediabetes in the United States, 2011. 2011. Available at: https://www.cdc.gov/diabetes/pubs/pdf/ndfs_2011.pdf. Accessed April 29, 2017.
12. Menke A, Casagrande S, Geiss L, et al. Prevalence of and trends in diabetes among adults in the United States, 1988-2012. JAMA 2015;314(10):1021–9.
13. Boyle JP, Thompson TJ, Gregg EW, et al. Projection of the year 2050 burden of diabetes in the US adult population: dynamic modeling of incidence, mortality, and prediabetes prevalence. Popul Health Metr 2010;8(1):29.
14. Fonseca V. Clinical diabetes. Philadelphia: Elsevier; 2006.
15. Burant CF, Young LA, editors. Medical management of T2DM. 7th edition. Alexandria (VA): American Diabetes Association; 2012.
16. Kaur J. A comprehensive review on metabolic syndrome. Cardiol Res Pract 2014; 2014:943162.
17. Herder C, Færch K, Carstensen-Kirberg M, et al. Biomarkers of subclinical inflammation and increases in glycaemia, insulin resistance and beta-cell function in non-diabetic individuals: the Whitehall II Study. Eur J Endocrinol 2016;175(5):367–77.
18. den Biggelaar LJ, Sep SJ, Eussen SJ, et al. Discriminatory ability of simple OGTT-based beta cell function indices for prediction of prediabetes and T2DM: the CODAM study. Diabetologia 2017;60(3):432–41.
19. Gregg EW, Geiss L, Zhang P, et al. Implications of risk stratification for diabetes prevention: the case of hemoglobin A1c. Am J Prev Med 2013;44(4):S375–80.
20. Salpeter SR, Buckley NS, Kahn JA, et al. Meta-analysis: metformin treatment in persons at risk for diabetes mellitus. Am J Med 2008;121(2):149–57.e2.
21. Bellamy L, Casas J-P, Hingorani AD, et al. T2DM mellitus after gestational diabetes: a systematic review and meta-analysis. Lancet 2009;373(9677):1773–9.
22. Kim C, Newton KM, Knopp RH. Gestational diabetes and the incidence of T2DM. Diabetes Care 2002;25(10):1862–8.
23. Translation NCfCDPaHPDoD. In: Test CPS, editor: Centers for Disease Control and Prevention. Available at: https://www.cdc.gov/diabetes/prevention/pdf/prediabetestest.pdf. Accessed April 29, 2017.
24. Division of Nutrition PA, and Obesity, National Center for Chronic Disease Prevention and Health Promotion. About Child & Teen BMI. 2015. Available at: https://

www.cdc.gov/healthyweight/assessing/bmi/childrens_bmi/about_childrens_bmi. html. Accessed May 13, 2017.

25. Centers for Disease Control and Prevention. Awareness of prediabetes–United States, 2005-2010. MMWR Morb Mortal Wkly Rep 2013;62(11):209.

26. Grossmann V, Schmitt VH, Zeller T, et al. Profile of the immune and inflammatory response in individuals with prediabetes and T2DM. Diabetes Care 2015;38(7): 1356–64.

27. Sörensen BM, Houben AJ, Berendschot TT, et al. Prediabetes and T2DM are associated with generalized microvascular dysfunction: clinical perspective. Circulation 2016;134(18):1339–52.

28. Sullivan M. Brain atropy. Clinical endocrinology news, vol. 11. Parsippany (NJ): Frontline Medical Communications; 2016. p. 1–6. Available at: http://www.mdedge.com/clinicalendocrinologynews/article/113729/diabetes/brain-atrophy-already-evident-patients-prediabetes. Accessed September 14, 2016.

29. Ford ES, Zhao G, Li C. Pre-diabetes and the risk for cardiovascular disease. J Am Coll Cardiol 2010;55(13):1310–7.

30. National Center for Health Statistics. Health, United States, 2015: with special feature on racial and ethnic health disparities. 2015 edition. Hyattsville (MD): US Department of Health and Human Services Centers for Disease Control and Prevention National Center for Health Statistics; 2015.

31. Gong Q, Zhang P, Wang J, et al. Changes in mortality in people with IGT before and after the onset of diabetes during the 23-year follow-up of the Da Qing Diabetes Prevention Study. Diabetes Care 2016;39(9):1550–5.

32. Li G, Hu Y, Yang W, et al. Effects of insulin resistance and insulin secretion on the efficacy of interventions to retard development of T2DM mellitus: the DA Qing IGT and Diabetes Study. Diabetes Res Clin Pract 2002;58(3):193–200.

33. Diabetes Prevention Program (DPP) Research Group. The diabetes prevention program (DPP): description of lifestyle intervention. Diabetes Care 2002;25(12): 2165–71.

34. Ghody P, Shikha D, Karam J, et al. Identifying prediabetes–Is it beneficial in the long run? Maturitas 2015;81(2):282–6.

35. Lindström J, Peltonen M, Eriksson J, et al. Improved lifestyle and decreased diabetes risk over 13 years: long-term follow-up of the randomised Finnish Diabetes Prevention Study (DPS). Diabetologia 2013;56(2):284–93.

36. Beavers KM, Case LD, Blackwell CS, et al. Effects of weight regain following intentional weight loss on glucoregulatory function in overweight and obese adults with pre-diabetes. Obes Res Clin Pract 2015;9(3):266–73.

37. Tuomilehto J, Lindström J, Eriksson JG, et al. Prevention of T2DM mellitus by changes in lifestyle among subjects with impaired glucose tolerance. N Engl J Med 2001;344(18):1343–50.

38. Franz MJ, Boucher JL, Rutten-Ramos S, et al. Lifestyle weight-loss intervention outcomes in overweight and obese adults with T2DM: a systematic review and meta-analysis of randomized clinical trials. J Acad Nutr Diet 2015;115(9): 1447–63.

39. Roglic G. WHO Global report on diabetes: a summary. Int J Noncommun Dis 2016;1(1):3.

40. Division of Nutrition, Physical Activity, and Obesity, National Center for Chronic Disease Prevention and Health Promotion. Measuring physical activity intensity. 2015. Available at: https://www.cdc.gov/physicalactivity/basics/measuring/. Accessed May 13, 2017.

41. Diabetes Prevention Program Research Group. 10-year follow-up of diabetes incidence and weight loss in the Diabetes Prevention Program Outcomes Study. Lancet 2009;374(9702):1677–86.
42. Kim SH, Abbasi F, Lamendola C, et al. Benefits of liraglutide treatment in overweight and obese older individuals with prediabetes. Diabetes Care 2013; 36(10):3276–82.
43. Chiasson J-L, Josse RG, Gomis R, et al. Acarbose for prevention of T2DM mellitus: the STOP-NIDDM randomised trial. Lancet 2002;359(9323):2072–7.
44. DeFronzo RA, Tripathy D, Schwenke DC, et al. Prevention of diabetes with pioglitazone in ACT NOW. Diabetes 2013;62(11):3920–6.
45. Torgerson JS, Hauptman J, Boldrin MN, et al. Xenical in the prevention of diabetes in obese subjects (XENDOS) study. Diabetes Care 2004;27(1):155–61.
46. Pamidi S, Wroblewski K, Stepien M, et al. Eight hours of nightly continuous positive airway pressure treatment of obstructive sleep apnea improves glucose metabolism in patients with prediabetes. A randomized controlled trial. Am J Respir Crit Care Med 2015;192(1):96–105.
47. Centers for Disease Control and Prevention. National Diabetes Prevention Program. Available at: https://www.cdc.gov/diabetes/prevention/index.html. Accessed May 25, 2017.
48. National Institute of Diabetes and Digestive and Kidney Diseases. Available at: https://www.niddk.nih.gov/health-information/health-communication-programs/ndep/health-care-professionals/game-plan/Pages/index.aspx. Accessed May 25, 2017.
49. National Institute of Diabetes and Digestive and Kidney Diseases. Your game plan to prevent T2DM. 2017. Available at: https://www.niddk.nih.gov/health-information/diabetes/overview/preventing-type-2-diabetes/game-plan. Accessed May 25, 2017.
50. National Institute of Diabetes and Digestive and Kidney Diseases. NIDDK Publications Catalog: National Diabetes Education Program (NDEP) list of materials. Available at: https://catalog.niddk.nih.gov/Catalog/ndep.cfm. Accessed May 25, 2017.

Therapeutic Lifestyle Changes for Diabetes Mellitus

Celia Levesque, RN, MSN, CNS-BC, NP-C, CDE, BC-ADM*

KEYWORDS

- Diabetes mellitus • Medical nutrition therapy • Physical activity • Smoking cessation
- Diabetes distress • Diabetes self-management education
- Diabetes self-management support

KEY POINTS

- Diabetes mellitus is a common disease that carries a heavy burden psychologically, physically, and financially.
- Diabetes is a largely self-managed disease; however, the patient often is uninformed or receives the wrong information from friends, relatives, and media.
- Therapeutic lifestyle management is fundamental to meet glycemic targets and other diabetes-related health targets, such as blood pressure and lipids.
- Diabetes distress is different from other psychological disorders, and it can adversely affect diabetes outcomes.

INTRODUCTION

Diabetes mellitus is a chronic disease affecting more than 29 million Americans. An additional 86 million Americans have prediabetes.[1] Therapeutic lifestyle changes improve prediabetes and diabetes. Managing diabetes requires frequent decisions on a daily basis, which can be overwhelming, often causing patients to feel helpless and hopeless. In addition, patients often get misinformation from friends, relatives, and the media/Internet on how to best manage diabetes. This article discusses therapeutic lifestyle changes based on current standards of care.

Disclosure Statement: There are no commercial or financial conflicts of interest.
Department of Endocrine Neoplasia and Hormonal Disorders, MD Anderson Cancer Center, 1515 Holcomb Boulevard, Houston, TX 77030, USA
* 14726 Leighwood Creek Lane, Humble, TX 77396.
E-mail address: clevesqu@mdanderson.org

Nurs Clin N Am 52 (2017) 679–692
http://dx.doi.org/10.1016/j.cnur.2017.07.012
0029-6465/17/© 2017 Elsevier Inc. All rights reserved.
nursing.theclinics.com

DIABETES SELF-MANAGEMENT EDUCATION AND DIABETES SELF-MANAGEMENT SUPPORT

Diabetes self-management education and diabetes self-management support (DSME/S) helps to empower patients with diabetes to make intelligent decisions by providing the knowledge and skills to manage blood glucose and other diabetes-related comorbid conditions, such as hyperlipidemia and hypertension.[2] A team of health professionals provide the services but it is important that the patient and his or her significant others are at the center of the team because shared decision making is crucial to clinical, psychosocial, and behavioral outcomes.[3] Organizations including the American Association of Diabetes Educators, American Diabetes Association, American College of Endocrinology, and American Association of Clinical Endocrinology support the premise that all individuals with diabetes should receive DSME/S by a team of trained specialists.[2,4,5]

DSME/S programs have been shown to reduce the readmission rate of diabetes patients with poor glycemic control. A retrospective study of 2265 patients with poorly controlled diabetes with hemoglobin A_{1c} (HbA_{1c}) greater than 9% and hospitalized between years 2008 and 2010 showed that patients who received inpatient diabetes education had a significantly lower all-cause hospital readmission rate.[6] Therapeutic lifestyle changes are difficult. A study compared lifestyle behaviors of patients with newly diagnosed type 2 diabetes mellitus (T2DM) with those without diabetes.[7] The participants completed an extensive survey that included demographics, current health status, and lifestyle behaviors. The authors reported that patients with T2DM had lost significantly more weight, were less likely to reduce vegetable intake, and were more likely to quit smoking compared with those without a diagnosis of T2DM.[7]

Four key times are identified when patients with diabetes need DSME/S[2,4,8]:

- At the time of diagnosis
- Annually for an educational needs assessment/teaching
- When new issues occur, such as
  - New diabetes-related complications
  - Changes in glycemic control
  - Emotional factors
  - Physical or mental inability to care for self
- When transitions in care occur

The diabetes education provided is based on an educational assessment, which includes the following[2,4,5]:

- Current knowledge
- Health beliefs
- Cultural influences
- Comorbid conditions
- Literacy (number and words)
- Financial status
- Support from significant others

Based on the assessment, the education at diagnosis should begin with the basics of self-care and build from there. The basics include[2,4,5]

- Treatment goals
- Blood glucose monitoring
- Meal planning
- Physical activity

- Medication management
- Prevention of acute complications
- Foot care
- Smoking cessation if needed

A subsequent educational assessment should be performed annually, when new issues arise, and during periods of transition. The assessment should include[2,4,5]

- Reviewing treatment goals
- Assessing current health maintenance habits
- Assessing changes in financial status and support from significant others
- Assessing the ability of the patient to care for self
- Assessing the level of psychological distress/coping with diabetes self-care
- Providing support and education based on the needs assessment
- Involving significant others in the care of the patient if needed

DIABETES TREATMENT TARGETS

Treatment targets should be individualized depending on factors including

- Current age
- Duration of diabetes
- Risk of hypoglycemia

Table 1
Treatment targets for diabetes mellitus

Premeal BG, mg/dL	Excellent: <110 Acceptable: <130	
Postprandial BG, mg/dL	Excellent: <140 Acceptable: <180	
HbA$_{1c}$	<7% if no hypoglycemia	
Weight	Body mass index <25 5%–10% weight reduction in overweight or obese patients	
Activity	150 min/wk moderately intense Strength training 2–3 times/wk	
Sleep	6–9 h per night	
Tobacco use	None	
Blood pressure	<140/90 mm Hg Lower goal if high-risk cardiovascular disease and can be achieved without excessive treatment	
Lipids	*High-risk patients*	*Very high risk*
LDL-C, mg/dL	<100	<70
Non-HDL-C, mg/dL	<130	<100
Triglycerides, mg/dL	<150	<150
TC/HDL-C	<3.5	<3
Apo B, mg/dL	<90	<80
LDL-P, mmol/L	<1200	<1000

Drink equivalent: 5 ounces wine, 1.5 ounce distilled spirits, 12 ounces beer.[4,5]
Abbreviations: Apo B, apolipoprotein B; BG, blood glucose; HDL-C, high-density lipoprotein cholesterol; LDL-C, low-density lipoprotein cholesterol; LDL-P, low-density lipoprotein particle; TC, total cholesterol.

- Presence of comorbid conditions
- Life expectancy
- Motivation/patient desire
- Capability of caring for self
- Social support
- Financial situation

Table 2
Nutrition recommendations for diabetes mellitus

Topic	Recommendation

Calories	• Calorie intake to meet desirable weight
	• 5%–10% weight loss in overweight and obese patients using
	   ○ 500–750 calorie/d deficit
	   ○ 1200–1500 calories/d in women
	   ○ 1500–1800 calories/d in men
	• Intervention programs to help patients meet goals are encouraged

Distribution of macronutrients	No single ideal dietary distribution of calories between carbohydrate, protein, and fat. Individualize the percent distribution while maintaining the desired caloric intake.
Protein	In patients with T2DM, protein may induce insulin secretion so protein should not be consumed to prevent or treat hypoglycemia.
Fat	Monounsaturated fats and foods containing long-chain omega-3 fatty acids (found in fatty fish) may lower cardiovascular risk; however, there is no evidence to support taking over-the-counter fish oil supplements.
Carbohydrate	Carbohydrate intake recommendations should be made based on the individual's blood glucose response. Refined carbohydrates should be limited; whole grains, legumes, vegetables, and fruits are a better choice. Using whole-grain was not associated with improved glycemic control; however, it did show a reduction in cardiovascular disease mortality. Individuals with T1DM using a basal-bolus insulin program or insulin pump should use an insulin/carbohydrate ratio to determine prandial insulin doses. For patients not on a basal-bolus insulin program, a consistent carbohydrate diet is recommended to minimize wide fluctuations in blood glucose.
Sodium	The recommendations are the same as for the general population, <2300 mg/d. A lower sodium intake may be beneficial in treating hypertension.
Alcohol	If the individual does not drink, do not recommend starting. Alcohol may contribute to the development of hypoglycemia if the individual is taking insulin, or an insulin secretagogue; provide education on the prevention and treatment of hypoglycemia. Alcohol intake should be limited to a maximum of 1 drink equivalent per day for adult women and 2 drink equivalents per day in men. The following is a drink equivalents: • 12 ounces beer (5% alcohol) • 5 ounces wine • 1.5 ounces distilled spirits (40% alcohol)
Nonnutritive sweeteners	Nonnutritive sweeteners do not impact the blood glucose and may be used as desired. The patient needs to be educated that products that are labeled as "sugar free" may not be calorie free or carbohydrate free. Products that are labeled as 0 calories may be consumed as desired.
Supplements	There are no studies supporting the use of supplements to improve diabetes outcomes. Patients that are found to have deficiencies may be supplemented, such as in vitamin B_{12} and D deficiencies.

The patient needs to be in agreement with the treatment targets and educated on ways to achieve targets. **Table 1** contains the recommended treatment targets for diabetes mellitus.[4]

NUTRITION THERAPY RECOMMENDATIONS FOR DIABETES MELLITUS

Currently, there is no such thing as a "diabetic diet." Caloric intake rather than percent macronutrients (carbohydrate, fat, and protein) is the main cause of weight so medical nutrition therapy is individualized to the patient to meet weight and nutritional goals. The goals of nutrition therapy for adults with diabetes include (1) promotion of healthy eating patterns; (2) meet nutritional needs based on a comprehensive assessment of the individual's food preferences, access to food, culture, willingness, ability, and barriers to make any needed changes; and (3) provide practical advice on healthy eating patterns rather than focusing on individual macronutrients, micronutrients, or certain foods.[4]

In general the meal plan that is encouraged includes a primarily plant-based diet. The fat that is consumed should be polyunsaturated and monounsaturated fatty acids with limited intake of saturated fatty acids and avoidance of *trans* fat. Patients who are overweight with a body mass index (BMI) of 25 to 29.9 or obese with a BMI of 30 or greater should strive to reduce weight by 5% to 10%.[5] Sustained weigh loss in patients with T2DM has been shown to reduce the need for diabetes medications, especially early in the disease process before irreversible severe β-cell dysfunction occurs[4] **(Table 2)**.

Mediterranean Diet

Many studies show that the Mediterranean diet is associated with a 30% reduction of developing T2DM. Salas-Salvado and coworkers[9] conducted a meta-analysis looking at the effects of the Mediterranean diet on T2DM and metabolic syndrome and found that with increased use of the Mediterranean diet there was a reduction in the development of T2DM and a reduction of cardiovascular risk in patients with T2DM. The combination of eating high-quality foods including fruits, vegetables, whole grains, olive oil, and seafood may reduce inflammation and insulin resistance and improve endothelial function[10] **(Fig. 1)**.

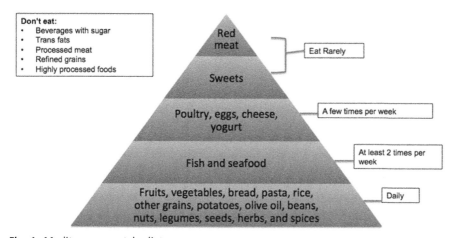

Fig. 1. Mediterranean-style diet.

Dietary Approaches to Stop Hypertension Diet

The Dietary Approaches to Stop Hypertension Diet (**Fig. 2**) is used in patients with diabetes to improve blood pressure, insulin resistance, hyperlipidemia, and weight. This diet is low in saturated fat, total fat, sodium (<2300 mg/day), and cholesterol. It is high in potassium, calcium, magnesium, fiber, and protein. Foods including whole grains, low-fat dairy products, fruits (not juices), vegetables, poultry, fish, seafood, eggs, legumes, and nuts are encouraged. High-fat meats, full-fat dairy products, tropical oils, and sugar-containing foods and beverages are discouraged.[11]

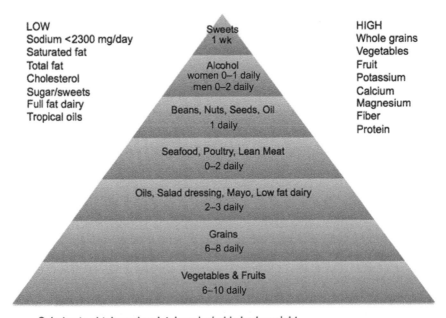

LOW
Sodium <2300 mg/day
Saturated fat
Total fat
Cholesterol
Sugar/sweets
Full fat dairy
Tropical oils

Sweets
1 wk

Alcohol
women 0–1 daily
men 0–2 daily

Beans, Nuts, Seeds, Oil
1 daily

Seafood, Poultry, Lean Meat
0–2 daily

Oils, Salad dressing, Mayo, Low fat dairy
2–3 daily

Grains
6–8 daily

Vegetables & Fruits
6–10 daily

HIGH
Whole grains
Vegetables
Fruit
Potassium
Calcium
Magnesium
Fiber
Protein

Calories to obtain and maintain a desirable body weight

Fig. 2. Dietary Approaches to Stop Hypertension Diet.

The Plate Method

Many patients with diabetes find meal planning for diabetes confusing and because the recommendations for healthy eating is the same for all people, with or without diabetes. The MyPlate method, based on the food pyramid, is an easy way to teach healthy eating. The US Department of Agriculture has a Web site devoted to the MyPlate method containing free online tools including a BMI calculator, free print materials including sample menus, and videos.[12] The author, along with a group of professionals at M.D. Anderson Cancer Center, developed a plastic reusable placemat for patients with diabetes that is based on the plate method (**Fig. 3**). The placemat contains a 9-inch picture of a plate (the actual size of the plate recommended for the patient to use). Half of the plate contains nonstarchy vegetables, one-quarter of the plate is starch, and one-quarter of the plate is protein. The patient may add fruit and milk to the meal depending on the calorie recommendations. The front of the placemat also includes instructions for label reading. The back of the placemat contains a serving size guide, and food groups with serving sizes.

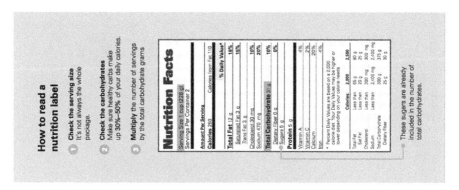

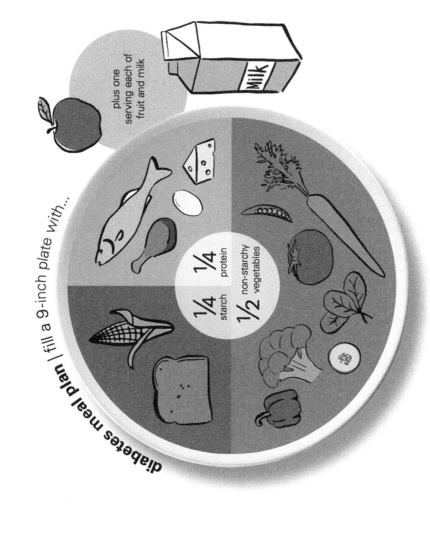

Fig. 3. Diabetes placemat.

Meat or protein
0 carbohydrate

Limit to 3–4 oz. per meal

Beef	1 oz.
Buffalo	1 oz.
Cheese	1 oz.
Chicken	1 oz.
Cornish hen	1 oz.
Cottage cheese	¼ cup
Duck	1 oz.
Egg	1
Egg white	2
Fish	1 oz.
Ham	1 oz.
Hot dog	1 oz.
Kidney	1 oz.
Lamb	1 oz.
Liver	1 oz.
Oysters	6
Parmesan (grated)	2 tbsp
Peanut butter	1 tbsp
Pork	1 oz.
Ricotta	2 oz. or ¼ cup
Sausage	1 oz.
Turkey	1 oz.
Veal	1 oz.

Milk
12 grams of carbohydrate

It's better to choose low-fat milk

Milk	1 cup
Soy milk	1 cup
Buttermilk	1 cup
Evaporated milk	½ cup
Dry milk	⅓ cup
Yogurt (plain)	¾ cup

Vegetables
5 grams of carbohydrate

1 cup raw or ½ cup cooked

Artichoke
Artichoke hearts
Asparagus
Beans (green, wax, etc.)
Bean sprouts
Beets
Brussels sprouts
Cabbage
Cauliflower
Celery
Cucumber
Eggplant
Greens
Green onions
Leeks
Mushrooms
Okra
Onion
Peppers
Radishes
Salad greens
Sauerkraut
Spinach
Summer squash
Tomato
Tomato sauce
Tomato juice
Watercress
Zucchini

Fruit
15 grams of carbohydrate

Avoid fruit juice

Apple	2 inch
Applesauce	½ cup
Apricots	4 small
Banana	1 small (4-inch)
Blackberries	¾ cup
Blueberries	¾ cup
Cantaloupe	⅓ of whole or 1 cup cubed
Cherries	12
Figs	2 medium
Fruit cocktail	½ cup
Grapefruit	½
Grapes (medium)	15
Honeydew	1 cup cubed
Kiwi large	1
Mandarin orange	¾ cup
Mango	½ cup
Nectarine	1 small
Orange	1 small
Peach	1 medium
Pear	1 small
Pineapple	¾ cup raw
Pineapple	½ cup canned
Plums	2 small
Raspberries	1 cup
Strawberries (whole)	1¼ cup
Tangerine	2 small
Watermelon	1¼ cup

Starch
15 grams of carbohydrate

Measure starch portions

Animal cracker	8
Baked beans	⅓ cup
Bagel	¼ of bagel
Beans	½ cup
Biscuit	2½ inch
Bread	1 slice
Bread (40 cal)	2 slices
Cereal	½ cup
Chips	1 oz
Corn	½ cup
Cornbread	2-inch
Crackers	5-6
English muffin	1/2
French fries	16
Graham cracker	3 squares
Granola	¼ cup
Grits	½ cup
Hamburger bun or hot dog bun	½
Lentils	½ cup
Lima beans	⅔ cup
Muffin	small
Noodles	½ cup
Pancake/ waffle	4-inch
Pasta	⅓ cup
Peas	½ cup
Pita	½
Popcorn (cooked)	3 cups
Potato (white or sweet)	½ cup
Rice (cooked)	⅓ cup
Roll	1 oz.
Winter squash	1 cup
Tortilla	6 inch

Fat
0 carbohydrate

Almonds	6
Avocado	⅛
Bacon	1 slice
Butter	1 tsp
Chitterlings	½ oz.
Coconut	2 tbsp
Cream (half & half)	2 tbsp
Cream (heavy)	1 tbsp
Cream cheese	1 tbsp
Cream cheese (light)	2 tbsp
Margarine	1 tsp
Margarine (reduced fat)	1 tbsp
Mayonnaise	1 tsp
Oil	1 tsp
Olives black	8 large
Olive green	10 large
Salt pork	¼ oz.
Salad dressing	1 tbsp
Salad dressing (reduced fat)	2 tbsp
Shortening	1 tsp
Sour cream	2 tbsp
Sour cream (light)	3 tbsp

Free Foods
Unlimited

Bouillon or broth
Calorie-free beverages
Mustard
Lemon juice
Lime juice
Horseradish
Sugar substitute
Sugar free gelatin
Sugar free gum
Jalapeño
Pico de gallo

Free Foods
Limited to 1 per meal

Catsup	1 tbsp
Cocoa powder (unsweetened)	1 tbsp
Hard candy (sugar-free)	1 piece
Jam/jelly (sugar-free)	2 tsp
Pancake syrup (sugar-free)	2 tbsp
Pickles	1½ large
Mayonnaise (reduced fat)	1 tbsp

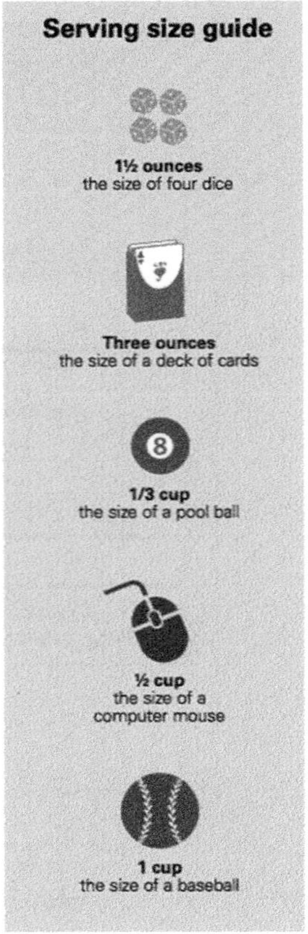
Serving size guide
1½ ounces
the size of four dice
Three ounces
the size of a deck of cards
8
1/3 cup
the size of a pool ball
½ cup
the size of a computer mouse
1 cup
the size of a baseball

Fig. 3. (*continued*).

Vegetarian Diets

Vegetarians have a lower prevalence of T2DM compared with nonvegetarians. In patients with T2DM, a plant-based diet improved glycemic control, reduced calorie consumption and weight, reduced HbA_{1c}, and reduced need for diabetes medications.[13] There are a variety of vegetarian-type diets (**Table 3**).

Vegan diets are associated with improvement in neuropathy pain, a reduction of the decline of kidney function in patients with advanced chronic kidney disease, and a reduction of cardiovascular risk. On the down side, the vegetarian diets are associated with a higher risk for B_{12} deficiency, low vitamin D, low calcium, and low iron. People on a vegetarian diet consume less eicosapentaenoic acid and docosahexaenoic acid found in long-chain omega-3 fatty acids. These deficiencies increase the risk for retinopathy, neuropathy, bone fractures, and cardiovascular disease, so the patient should be monitored and treated for deficiencies.[13]

Ramadan

Fasting during Ramadan is mandatory for all healthy people of the Muslim faith who have reached puberty. It occurs during the ninth month of the Muslim calendar. Because Ramadan is based on the lunar calendar, it occurs 10 to 11 days earlier each year. Although people with serious illness are exempt from fasting, most patients with diabetes want to participate and can safely fast during Ramadan. During the fast, the observer must refrain from drinking, eating, smoking, taking oral medications, and having sexual relations from dawn until sunset. The time from dawn until sunset is different each day, and it differs geographically so the fasting period may be as long as 20 hours. The amount and types of foods eaten when the fast is broken is often different from the observer's usual eating pattern when not fasting. A large proportion of total daily caloric intake occurs soon after sunset. Sleep patterns are also changed. The observer may wake up before dawn to eat before starting the fast, then go back to sleep and arise later in the day. Many stay awake well past midnight. The total amount of sleep is reduced as well as rapid eye movement sleep. The reduced sleep causes changes in body temperature and cortisol, which can cause insulin resistance;

Table 3	
Characteristics of various types of vegetarian diets	
Type of Vegetarian Diet	**Characteristics of Diet**
Vegan/raw food vegan	No animal products including meat, honey, dairy, eggs, meat by-products (gelatin and meat broth)
Ovovegetarian	Consumes eggs Does not consume meat, meat by-products, gelatin and meat broth, dairy by-products
Lactovegetarian	Consumes dairy Does not consume meat, meat by-products, eggs, gelatin, and meat broth
Lacto-ovo-vegetarian	Consumes dairy and eggs Does not consume meat
Pollotarian	Consumes poultry, fowl, eggs, and dairy Does not consume red meat, fish, and seafood
Pescatarian	Consumes fish, seafood, eggs, dairy Does not consume red meat

however, after 12 hours of fasting, liver glycogen stores are reduced, insulin levels are low, and fatty acids are released so the overall effect on blood glucose is not significant in most patients. A study of 63 people observing Ramadan who wore a continuous glucose monitor showed that fasting did not significantly change glycemic control.[14] A small study found that with diabetes education, the HbA_{1c} levels and mean blood glucose levels did not significantly change before and after Ramadan, serum fructosamine levels after Ramadan were reduced by 10%, and hypoglycemia events declined.[15]

The major risks associated with fasting include diabetic ketoacidosis, hypoglycemia, hyperglycemia, and dehydration. The factors to determine risk include type of diabetes, current diabetes medications, risk and history of hypoglycemia, presence of comorbid conditions, and individual lifestyle situation.

Many providers do not have the basic knowledge to advise the patient on how to manage diabetes while fasting.[16] The American Diabetes Association published recommendations for managing diabetes during Ramadan in 2005. The recommendations were updated in 2010 and again in 2015 (**Table 4**).[17]

Diabetes education for patients observing Ramadan includes teaching the signs, symptoms, treatment, and prevention of hypoglycemia; blood glucose

Table 4
Assessment of risk for patients with diabetes observing Ramadan

Risk	Patient Characteristics
Very high risk Fasting not recommended	• T1DM • Recent history of severe hypoglycemia • HbA_{1c} >10% or average fasting/premeal blood glucose values >300 mg/dL • Recent history of diabetic ketoacidosis or hyperglycemic hyperosmolar state • Severe comorbid conditions, such as stage IV or V chronic kidney disease • Pregnancy • Acutely ill • Inability to care for self/presence of cognitive deficits
High risk May choose not to fast	• Use of insulin or a secretagogue, especially if living alone • HbA_{1c} 8%–10% or average fasting/premeal blood glucose 150–300 mg/dL • Significant microvascular and macrovascular complications, or having a condition that makes fasting hazardous • Age >75 y
Moderate risk May choose to fast with caution	• Healthy • HbA_{1c} <8% • Treated with diabetes medications with a low risk of hypoglycemia metformin, α-glucosidase inhibitors, pioglitazone, and/or incretin therapy short-acting insulin secretagogues
Low risk May choose to fast	• Healthy • HbA_{1c} <7% • Treated with lifestyle interventions only or diabetes medications with a low risk for hypoglycemia including metformin, α-glucosidase inhibitors, pioglitazone, and/or incretin therapy

Adapted from Ibrahim M, Al Magd MA, Annabi FA, et al. Recommendations for management of diabetes during Ramadan: update 2015. BMJ Open Diabetes Res Care 2015;3(1):e000108.

monitoring; recommendations for fluid and caloric intake when not fasting; when to break the fast (<70 or >250–300 mg/dL), and treatment changes after Ramadan is finished.[17]

Weight Loss Programs

Intensive weight-loss management programs are often only found in medical centers, so many are not able to access those programs. Less formal weight-loss programs that combine reduced calories and increased activity can also be effective. Portion-controlled meal replacement products have been found to be effective for overweight individuals with diabetes. A study of 100 participants with T2DM who had a BMI of 25 to 50 and a HbA1 of 6.5% or greater and less than 12% were randomized into one of two treatment groups: lifestyle intervention using a portion-controlled diet, or a nine-session group program of DSME. Both groups were prescribed the same caloric goals and physical activity. The study showed that the patient's in the portion-controlled diet group lost an average of 7.3 kg compared with 2.2 kg in the DSME group. The HbA_{1c} reduction in the portion-controlled diet group was 0.7% compared with 0.4% in the DSME group.[18]

PHYSICAL ACTIVITY RECOMMENDATIONS FOR DIABETES MELLITUS

Moderate to vigorous regular physical activity helps to reduce the risk of progression from prediabetes to T2DM, and in patients with T2DM it reduces the risk of cardiovascular disease, improves blood glucose, and reduces all-cause mortality. Although physical activity has not been shown to improve glycemic control in patients with T1DM, patients with T1DM should exercise to gain the same benefits as patients without diabetes.

Physical activity recommendations for patients with diabetes include the following[4]:

- Children and adolescents with diabetes should engage in 60 min/day in moderate- or vigorous-intensity aerobic activity and muscle-strengthening and bone-strengthening activity at least 3 d/wk.
- Adults with diabetes should engage in 150 minutes or more of moderate to vigorous physical activity per week.
- Adults with diabetes should engage in two to three sessions per week of resistance exercise on nonconsecutive days.
- Sedentary time should be limited to no longer than 30 minutes without moving.
- Flexibility training and balance training, such as yoga and tai chi, is recommended in older adults with diabetes.

Table 5 provides exercise precautions for patients with diabetes.

SMOKING CESSATION

Patients with diabetes who smoke or exposed to secondhand smoke have an increased risk for cardiovascular disease, premature death, and microvascular complications. A meta-analysis of 88 studies shows that active and passive smoking is associated with significantly increased risks of T2DM.[19] The American Diabetes Association recommends the following regarding nicotine use in patients with diabetes[4]:

- Assess patients at each visit for all forms of tobacco and e-cigarettes
- Recommend cessation for users of all forms of tobacco and e-cigarettes
- Nonsmokers should be advised to not use e-cigarettes; however, e-cigarettes may be beneficial in helping smokers to quit

Table 5
Exercise precautions for patients with diabetes

Precaution	Recommendation
Cardiovascular disease	• Routine screening for coronary or disease in patients with diabetes is not recommended. • Assess cardiovascular risk factors and be aware of a typical presentation of coronary artery disease in patients with diabetes. • High-risk patients should start with short periods of low-intensity exercise and increase very slowly.
Hypoglycemia	• Patients who take insulin or insulin secretagogues may develop hypoglycemia during or after exercise. Patients beginning an exercise program should check blood glucose levels before, during, and after exercise to assess their individual response to exercise. • If the pre-exercise blood glucose level is <100 mg/dL the individual may need to consume carbohydrate before exercise. • Carbohydrate may be needed during exercise depending on the intensity and duration.
Retinopathy	• In patients with severe nonproliferative diabetic retinopathy or proliferative diabetic retinopathy, vigorous-intensity aerobic or resistance exercise may be contraindicated because it may trigger a vitreous hemorrhage or retinal detachment. The patient should consult with an ophthalmologist before starting an intense exercise program.
Peripheral neuropathy	• Patients who have a decreased sensation to the feet and lower legs are at risk for skin breakdown and Charcot joint. • The patient should have a foot examination, which includes a monofilament check to assess feeling and the patient should acquire properly fitting shoes before starting an exercise program. • Patients should be instructed how to assess their feet daily. • Any patients with a foot injury or open sore should not engage in weight-bearing activities.
Autonomic neuropathy	• Autonomic neuropathy increases the risk for decreased cardiac responsiveness to exercise, postural hypotension, impaired thermal regulation, decreased papillary reaction causing impaired night vision, and hypoglycemia unawareness. • Cardiac evaluation before starting an exercise program is recommended.
Diabetic kidney disease	• There is no exercise restriction in patients with diabetic kidney disease. • Exercise may increase urinary albumin excretion; however, vigorous-intensity exercise has not been shown to increase progression of diabetic kidney disease.

- Patients should avoid second-hand smoke
- Smoking cessation treatments including pharmacologic and nonpharmacologic should be recommended based on patient preference, level of dependence, and history of relapse
- Counsel patients that weight gain after smoking cessation is less detrimental to the development of cardiovascular disease than smoking

PSYCHOLOGICAL DISTRESS IN PATIENTS WITH DIABETES

Patients with diabetes should be assessed for psychosocial issues, especially if the glycemic and other medical targets are not being met, or if a significant change has occurred in their health, work, or family life. The screening should include the following[4]:

- Feelings about their diabetes and/or diabetes-related complications
- Expectations for treatment and outcomes
- Resources available to assist the patient in the management of their diabetes
- Cognitive ability to care for self
- Any underlying distress including depression, anxiety, disordered eating, cognitive

The assessment can begin with general questions to see if further formal testing is needed. There are many validated tools to assess patients. Referral to a mental health specialist may be needed if

- The patient is not performing self-care after individualized diabetes education
- The patient is shown to have depression with a valid screening tool
- If the patient has an eating disorder or omits insulin to lose weight
- If the patient has an extreme fear of hypoglycemia
- If the patient has a serious mental illness complicating diabetes self-care
- Patients with repeated diabetic ketoacidosis
- If the patient has declining or impaired ability to perform diabetes self-care
- Before and after bariatric surgery

SUMMARY

Therapeutic lifestyle changes are fundamental to achieve treatment targets, minimize the use of diabetes medications, and reduce the risk of comorbid conditions and psychological distress. Diabetes education and support, provided by diabetes specialists, is vital to successful self-management of diabetes. The diabetes management plan should be based on a thorough assessment of patient needs. Adjustments in the plan are needed periodically to achieve treatment targets.

REFERENCES

1. Centers for Disease Control and Prevention. National diabetes statistics report: Estimates of diabetes and its burden in the United States, 2014. 2014. Available at: http://www.cdc.gov/diabetes/data/statistics/2014statisticsreport. html. Accessed May 15, 2017.
2. Powers MA, Bardsley J, Cypress M, et al. Diabetes self-management education and support in type 2 diabetes: a joint position statement of the American Diabetes Association, the American Association of Diabetes Educators, and the Academy of Nutrition and Dietetics. Diabetes Educ 2017;43(1):40–53.
3. Powers MA. If DSME were a pill, would you prescribe it? Diabetes Spectr 2017; 30(1):51–7.
4. Marathe PH, Gao HX, Close KL. American Diabetes Association standards of medical care in diabetes 2017. Diabetes Care 2017;40(S1):S1–135.
5. Garber A, Abrahamson M, Barzilay J, et al. AACE/ACE Consensus Statement Consensus statement by the American Association of Clinical Endocrinologists and American College of Endocrinology on the comprehensive type 2 diabetes management algorithm–2016 Executive Summary. 84. Endocr Pract 2016;22(1): 84–113.
6. Healy SJ, Black D, Harris C, et al. Inpatient diabetes education is associated with less frequent hospital readmission among patients with poor glycemic control. Diabetes care 2013;36(10):2960–7.
7. Chong S, Ding D, Byun R, et al. Lifestyle changes after a diagnosis of type 2 diabetes. Diabetes Spectr 2017;30(1):43–50.

8. Garber AJ, Abrahamson MJ, Barzilay JI, et al. Consensus statement by the American Association of Clinical Endocrinologists and American College of Endocrinology on the comprehensive type 2 diabetes management algorithm: 2016 executive summary. Endocr Pract 2016;22(1):84–113.

9. Salas-Salvadó J, Guasch-Ferré M, Lee C-H, et al. Protective effects of the Mediterranean diet on type 2 diabetes and metabolic syndrome. J Nutr 2016;146(4): 920S–7S.

10. Boucher JL. Mediterranean eating pattern. Circulation 2017;30(2):72–6.

11. Campbell AP. DASH eating plan: an eating pattern for diabetes management. Diabetes Spectr 2017;30(2):76–81.

12. United States Department of Agriculture. ChooseMyPlate.gov. 2017. Available at: https://www.choosemyplate.gov. Accessed May 15, 2017.

13. Pawlak R. Vegetarian diets in the prevention and management of diabetes and its complications. Diabetes Spectr 2017;30(2):82–8.

14. Lessan N, Hannoun Z, Hasan H, et al. Glucose excursions and glycaemic control during Ramadan fasting in diabetic patients: insights from continuous glucose monitoring (CGM). Diabetes Metab 2015;41(1):28–36.

15. Eid YM, Sahmoud SI, Abdelsalam MM, et al. Empowerment-based diabetes self-management education to maintain glycemic targets during Ramadan fasting in people with diabetes who are on conventional insulin: a feasibility study. Diabetes Spectr 2017;30(1):36–42.

16. Ahmedani MY, Hashmi BZ, Ulhaque MS. Ramadan and diabetes-knowledge, attitude and practices of general practitioners; a cross-sectional study. Pak J Med Sci 2016;32(4):846.

17. Ibrahim M, Al Magd MA, Annabi FA, et al. Recommendations for management of diabetes during Ramadan: update 2015. BMJ Open Diabetes Res Care 2015; 3(1):e000108.

18. Foster G, Wadden T, Lagrotte C, et al. A randomized comparison of a commercially available portion-controlled weight-loss intervention with a diabetes self-management education program. Nutr Diabetes 2013;3(3):e63.

19. Pan A, Wang Y, Talaei M, et al. Relation of active, passive, and quitting smoking with incident type 2 diabetes: a systematic review and meta-analysis. Lancet Diabetes Endocrinol 2015;3(12):958–67.

Printed and bound by CPI Group (UK) Ltd, Croydon, CR0 4YY

03/10/2024

01040507-0001